Strabismus Surgery

Ophthalmology Monographs

A series published by Oxford University Press in cooperation with the American Academy of Ophthalmology

Series Editor: Richard Parrish

1. *Retinal Detachment: Principles and Practice, second edition.*
   George F. Hilton, John B. McLean, and Daniel A. Brinton
2. *Electrophysiologic Testing in Disorders of the Retina, Optic Nerve, and Visual Pathway, second edition*
   Gerald Allen Fishman, David G. Birch, Graham E. Holder, and Mitchell G. Brigell
3. *Visual Fields: Examination and Interpretation, second edition*
   Thomas J. Walsh
4. *Glaucoma Surgery: Principles and Techniques, second edition*
   Edited by Robert N. Weinreb and Richard P. Mills
5. *Florescein and Indocyanine Green Angiography: Technique and Interpretation, second edition*
   Joseph W. Berkow, Robert W. Flower, David H. Orth, and James S. Kelley
7. *Cataract Surgery and Intraocular Lenses: A 21st-Century Perspective, second edition*
   Edited by Jerry G. Ford and Carol L. Karp
8. Volumes 1, 2, and 3. *Surgery of the Eyelid, Orbit and Lacrimal System*
   Edited by William B. Stewart
9. *Surgical Anatomy of the Ocular Adnexa: A Clinical Approach*
   David R. Jordan and Richard L. Anderson
10. *Optic Nerve Disorders*
    Edited by Lanning B. Kline
11. *Laser Photocoagulation of the Retina and Choroid* (with slide set)
    James C. Folk and José S. Pulido
12. *Low Vision Rehabilitation: Caring for the Whole Person*
    Edited by Donald C. Fletcher
13. *Glaucoma Medical Therapy: Principles and Management*
    Edited by Peter A. Netland and Robert C. Allen
14. *Diabetes and Ocular Disease: Past, Present, and Future Therapies*
    Edited by Harry W. Flynn and William E. Smiddy
15. *HIV/AIDS and the Eye: A Global Perspective*
    Emmett T. Cunningham and Rubens Belfort
16. *Corneal Dystrophies and Degenerations*
    Edited by Ming X. Wang
17. *Strabismus Surgery: Basic and Advanced Strategies*
    Edited by David A. Plager; written by Edward G. Buckley, David A. Plager, Michael X. Repka, and M. Edward Wilson; contributions by Marshall M. Parks and Gunter K. von Noorden

STRABISMUS SURGERY

Basic and Advanced Strategies

Edited by
DAVID A. PLAGER, MD

Written by
EDWARD G. BUCKLEY, MD
DAVID A. PLAGER, MD
MICHAEL X. REPKA, MD
M. EDWARD WILSON, MD

Contributions by
MARSHALL M. PARKS, MD
GUNTER K. VON NOORDEN, MD

Published by Oxford University Press
in cooperation with
the American Academy of Ophthalmology

OXFORD
UNIVERSITY PRESS
2004

OXFORD
UNIVERSITY PRESS

Oxford New York
Auckland Bangkok Buenos Aires Cape Town Chennai
Dar es Salaam Delhi Hong Kong Istanbul Karachi Kolkata
Kuala Lumpur Madrid Melbourne Mexico City Mumbai Nairobi
Sao Paulo Shanghai Taipei Tokyo Toronto

Published by Oxford University Press, Inc.
198 Madison Avenue, New York, New York 10016
www.oup.com

Library of Congress Cataloging-in-Publication Data
Strabismus surgery : basic and advanced strategies /
edited by David A. Plager ;
contributors, Edward G. Buckley, Michael X. Repka, M. Edward Wilson ;
commentators, Marshall M. Parks, Gunter K. Von Noorden.
p. ; cm. — (Ophthalmology monographs)
Includes bibliographical references and index.
ISBN 978-0-19-517023-8
1. Strabismus—Surgery.
I. Plager, David A. II. Buckley, Edward G. III. Repka, Michael X.
IV. Wilson, M. Edward.
V. Series.
[DNLM: 1. Ocular Motility Disorders—surgery.
2. Ophthalmologic Surgical Procedures—methods.
WW 410 S894 2004] RE771.S843 2004 617.7'62—dc22 2003019388

Foreword

Not long ago a prominent ophthalmologist asked the rhetorical question, "Strabismus? What is so difficult about it?" He answered himself saying, "When they're out, put them in; when they're in, put them out; when one's down, put it up. It's not that complicated." That flippant comment has been replaced by a more thoughtful, and deserved appreciation for the theory and practice of strabismology at the beginning of the twenty-first century.

It is universally agreed that strabismology is a legitimate sub-specialty in ophthalmology. This fact notwithstanding, a reasonable question remains, "Why another book dealing with this subject?" The answer to this question could start with a look backward. Strabismology in the United States has evolved in three eras, each with its own body of literature. The first started when Diffenbach in Germany, around the middle of the nineteenth century, described the first successful surgery for strabismus. The ability to treat misalignment of the eyes with surgery in effect inaugurated the sub-specialty of strabismology. This discipline became firmly established in the U.S. ophthalmologist's armamentarium during the remainder of the nineteenth century. This was heralded by the publication of numerous articles and several good books dealing with the subject.

The second era of the management of strabismus took place in the first half of the twentieth century. During these 50 years, surgical techniques were refined sometimes in extremely complex ways, anesthesia became safer, and results of surgery improved somewhat. More books were produced and the volume of literature also increased. During this period, strabismus was managed for the most part by the general ophthalmologist, only a few of whom also had a special interest in strabismus.

At the conclusion of World War II, the third era started. There was greater emphasis on sensory factors, further refinements, and in some ways simplification of surgical techniques, instrumentation was improved, synthetic absorbable sutures became available, and surgery was done on much younger children and even infants. All of this found the surgeon paying more attention to functional results. During this period the sub-specialty of strabismology became firmly established with fellowship programs, with even more books and journals available. Scientific meetings proliferated giving the opportunity for more meaningful communication between clinicians and also with colleagues in the basic sciences.

A careful look at *Strabismus Surgery: Basic and Advanced Strategies* completes the answer to the question, "Why another book on strabismus?" David A. Plager, himself an authority on strabismus management, along with the American Academy of Ophthalmology, recognized the need to write a book that provides an up-to-date systematic coverage of strategies for strabismus surgery as this subspecialty begins its fourth era. He does this with the help of three colleagues, Drs. Buckley, Repka, and Wilson, also authorities on strabismus management, who contribute in their particular areas of interest and expertise. Together they provide a concise, readable description of the best of the current techniques. Then, capitalizing on the freer communication of the current era, Dr. Plager asked each contributor to comment on the work of fellow authors. This fresh idea adds considerable value to the book by giving the reader options not available in a traditional text. This book also honors the existing body of knowledge concerning strabismus management by including the comments and critique of two masters of strabismology, Marshall M. Parks and Gunter K. von Noorden, men whose clinical careers spanned the entire third era of the field.

Strabismus Surgery: Basic and Advanced Strategies should be read by anyone serious about keeping current in the field of strabismus management. It honors the past, respects the present, and anticipates the future, answering the second question completely.

Eugene M. Helveston, MD

Preface

Surgical treatment of any pathology requires a combination of both the science and art of medicine. Few surgical disciplines require a greater measure of the art of medicine than the management of strabismus. Surgeons learn most of the science of strabismus from the printed literature or other didactic sources. Most of the art of strabismus is acquired through experience—either our own or that which has been passed on to us by those who learned before us. Paraphrasing philosopher George Santayana—those who fail to learn from the experience of others are condemned to repeat it.

The purpose of this book is to share much of the art (and science) of strabismus learned through the combined experience of the four authors. Each has benefited immeasurably by the opportunity to have learned directly from some of the greatest sources of strabismus surgery experience available in the second half of the twentieth century. Marshall M. Parks and the teaching faculty of the Washington, DC program directly trained two of the authors (DAP, MEW). Other luminaries whose own experience directly influenced one or more of the authors include Eugene Helveston, M.D., Robison Harley, M.D., David Guyton, M.D., David Friendly, M.D., John Flynn, M.D., F. Daryel Ellis, M.D., Joe Calhoun, M.D., and Judy Seaber, C.O.

Therefore, this book results from the combined experience of all of these surgeons and many others. The book is not intended to be an all inclusive scientific reference on strabismus—excellent sources of this such as Gunter von Noorden's *Binocular Vision and Ocular Motility* serve this need well. It is also not a beginning book for those unfamiliar with basic strabismus techniques. *Strabismus Surgery: Basic and Advanced Strategies* emphasizes clinical applicability, discussing surgical strategies and important examination techniques intended for anyone performing strabismus surgeries from the common horizontal muscle recession to the most complicated restrictive, paretic, or oblique muscle re-operation.

Each chapter includes that author's own biases and preferences as shaped by his experiences and influences. Each author, however, strove to present a balanced approach and to offer alternative workable strategies when appropriate. In order to help achieve overall balance, each of the other authors was asked to offer dissenting opinions about significant points that the reader will find interspersed throughout the book. Many of these conflicting or alternative approaches make for some of the most interesting reading. The book's value is further enhanced by the invited commentary of two of the giants of strabismology, Drs. Parks and von Noorden. Their contributions include helpful pearls of wisdom as well as several historical vignets that practitioners in this discipline will enjoy reading. I am most grateful to both of them for sharing their incomparable wealth of knowledge and experience, which is found in their commentary throughout this book.

I would also like to thank Sprague Eustis, M.D. and the monograph committee of the American Academy of Ophthalmology for planting the seed that initiated this project.

Indianapolis, Indiana D.A.P.

Contents

Contributors

Edward G. Buckley, M.D.
Professor of Ophthalmology & Pediatrics
Chief, Pediatric and Neuroophthalmology
Associate Dean for Undergraduate Medical Education
Duke University School of Medicine
Durham, NC

David A. Plager, M.D.
Professor of Ophthalmology
Director, Section of Pediatric Ophthalmology & Strabismus
Indiana University School of Medicine
Indianapolis, IN

Michael X. Repka, M.D.
Professor of Ophthalmology
Professor of Pediatrics
Johns Hopkins University School of Medicine
Baltimore, MD

M. Edward Wilson, M.D.
Pierre G. Jenkins Professor and Chairman
Department of Ophthalmology
Director, Albert Florens Storm Eye Institute
Medical University of South Carolina
Charleston, SC

COMMENTATORS

Gunter K. von Noorden, M.D.
Emeritus Professor of Ophthalmology
Longboat Key, FL

Marshall M. Parks, M.D.
Children's Hospital National Medical Center, Washington, DC
Professor of Ophthalmology
George Washington University Medical Center
Washington DC

Strabismus Surgery

1

Esotropic Deviations

MICHAEL X. REPKA

The signature disease of pediatric ophthalmology is esotropia. There are a number of subtypes, based on time of onset, presence of hypermetropic refractive error, and associated neurologic findings. These findings are not sufficient to adequately explain the actual cause of most cases of esotropia. The evaluation, medical and optical therapy, and surgery for correction of esodeviations of most causes is similar, except for those cases associated with extraocular muscle ductional deficits.

A number of statements can be made about esotropia. These will guide the clinician's approach to this clinical phenotype irrespective of cause.

1. The long-standing distinctions based on age of onset are imprecise and can be misleading.
2. Crossing of the eyes may be associated with accommodative effort associated with hypermetropia at any age. Significant hypermetropia should be corrected prior to surgical correction.
3. The younger the patient is at the time of realignment, the more likely the realignment will be successful when measured in terms of both motor alignment and sensory fusion. Presumably, this allows the developing cortex to establish binocular pathways more readily.
4. The shorter the period of constant misalignment, the more likely it is that the eyes will be realigned and resume binocular function. Presumably, the better outcome is made more likely because there has been less damage to the cortical mechanisms of binocularity from abnormal binocular experience.

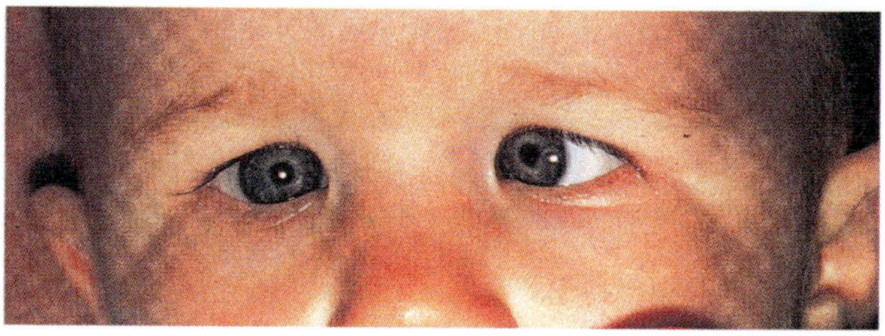

Figure 1–1. Infantile (early-onset) esotropia.

INFANTILE ESOTROPIA

The most recognizable, though not the most common, form of esotropia is infantile, or early-onset, esotropia (Fig. 1–1). Onset is typically within the first 6 months of life. Many authors have termed this esotropic deviation *congenital esotropia*, although only a few infants are born with the condition. (In this chapter, the term *infantile esotropia* is used.) Initially, the deviation may be small and intermittent, but it increases over the first year of life in both frequency and magnitude until it becomes constant and typically large-angle: 35 prism diopters (Δ) or more.

The initial ophthalmologic examination should include at least a qualitative assessment of visual acuity, pupillary examination, primary-position alignment, testing of ductions, and ophthalmoscopy. The last should include visualization of at least the optic disc and macula. This serves to eliminate important retinal and optic nerve diseases as the cause of the deviation. In addition, at least one cycloplegic refraction is necessary. These infants typically have small-magnitude hypermetropia, less than +2.50 diopters (D).

COMMENT

Marshall M. Parks, MD

The initial ophthalmologic visit should include a careful family history regarding strabismus in other family members. Even better is a casual assessment of any family member accompanying the patient. Primary monofixation syndrome occurs 11 times more frequently among first-order relatives of infantile esotropia patients than among the normal population. The second most frequently expressed feature of this prevalent genetic disorder is esotropia. Other close family members without strabismus or anisometropia, who have only the primary monofixation syndrome, appear to transmit the infantile esotropia component to their progeny at approximately the same rate as parents who have the infantile esotropia.

COMMENT

Gunter K. von Noorden, MD

In our experience, a hypermetropia of 2.00 D or less occurred in only 57% of 408 cases. In Costenbader's series of 500 cases, this was true in only 46%. It is our impression that the distribution of refractive errors in patients with infantile esotropia is not different from that in a nonstrabismic population.

Associated Findings. Early-onset strabismus is associated with overaction of the inferior oblique muscles, latent nystagmus, amblyopia, and the dissociated strabismus complex. (For a detailed discussion of the last, see Chapter 4, "Dissociated Deviations.") These features typically are not present at the outset of the esotropia. The prevalence of each of these signs increases over the first few years of life. Most patients develop them after the initial treatment of the esotropia has been successfully completed. Although most often seen with early-onset esotropia, they also occur with both exotropia and acquired esotropia.

Latent nystagmus is conjugate and binocular. The direction of eye movements on cover testing is diagnostic. The viewing eye drifts nasally (slow phase), while the refixation (fast) phase is directed temporally. When the cover is moved to the fellow eye, the slow phase shifts direction and again the viewing eye moves toward the nose. No other form of nystagmus shifts direction with a change of fixation.

Inferior oblique overaction (IOOA) is usually bilateral and symmetric. It is characterized by overelevation of the eye in adduction. Examination of the fundus may demonstrate excyclotorsion, helping to confirm the inferior oblique muscle overaction as the cause of the upshoot.

The dissociated strabismus complex may include vertical, horizontal, and torsional deviations, although a dissociated vertical deviation (DVD) is the most prominent form. It may be difficult to differentiate DVD from IOOA, especially since they frequently coexist. The presence of true IOOA can be established by having the patient fixate with one eye in adduction. If the abducted eye is hypotropic, the patient's vertical deviation is due to IOOA. If the abducted eye is hypertropic or level with the fixating eye, the deviation is due to DVD. If the refixating downward movement of the adducted eye is greater in magnitude than the upward refixation saccade of the abducting eye, the patient has DVD superimposed on IOOA. This last instance may be the most common.

Nonsurgical Treatment. Medical therapy for early-onset esotropia is limited to the use of occlusion for the prevention and treatment of amblyopia. Most practitioners prefer to intervene when there is a fixation preference, prescribing occlusion to the preferred eye for varying periods of time per day. This author prefers to use no more than 6 hours per day of occlusion during the first 6 months of life. Parents are taught how to identify the fixating eye and then adjust the patching duration to maintain some alternation. It is not necessary to extinguish all fixation preference, as this will likely overtreat any amblyopia present.

COMMENT
Edward G. Buckley, MD

I prefer days of patching as opposed to hours per day. It is much easier to simply place a patch on an eye for a day than it is to remember how long the patch has been on for any given day. Thus, it is far easier to have alternate-day patching than to patch one eye 50% of the time each day. I also prefer to minimize the time that the patient is *not* patched during the treatment phase. Allowing the child to select a preferred eye and actively suppress the other seems counterproductive.

A planned program of alternate-eye occlusion has been suggested for all patients with esotropia from the time of diagnosis until the eyes are realigned. These infants wear a patch every waking hour on one or the other eye. The hypothesis is that the maintenance of the monocular state will prevent development of suppression or abnormal binocular interaction. The utility of this approach is controversial.

COMMENT
Marshall M. Parks, MD

The concept that full-time alternate occlusion, from the time of diagnosis of infantile esotropia until the eyes are aligned, is beneficial by preventing development of suppression impresses me as totally fallacious. Suppression is an adaptation of the normal binocular vision cortex designed to eliminate the annoyance of diplopia that results in a patient with normal retinal correspondence (NRC) fusion after the onset of strabismus. The infant with a large-angle constant esotropia is unable to develop binocular vision reflexes until the eyes are aligned. The adaptations of normal binocular vision are not able to develop until normal binocular vision has first developed. Therefore, my opinion is that the program of alternate constant occlusion prior to surgical alignment is useless and disturbing to both the parents and their esotropic child.

Antiaccommodative therapy is considered for only a few of these infants. Patients with hypermetropia greater than +2.25 D should undergo a trial of hypermetropic correction. Even a few patients with modest hypermetropia may respond to this therapy. Those with greater hypermetropia (greater than +3.00 D) are more likely to respond to spectacle therapy. These patients with unusually early-onset refractive esotropia must be distinguished from those who have infantile esotropia with a coincidental high hyperopic refractive error. When glasses are prescribed, a 30-day trial of the spectacles is sufficient prior to surgical correction. An office trial may be inconclusive, as the accommodative effort is unlikely to relax in such a brief interval. Some children may require a short course of topical atropine, 1% once daily in each eye for several days, to relax tonic accommodation.

COMMENT
Edward G. Buckley, MD

In large-angle infantile esotropia patients, I generally do not use spectacle correction for hyperopia less than 3.00 D. This strategy changes if there is a residual deviation after strabismus surgery. In that circumstance, I think any hyperopia greater than 3.00 D should be corrected before recommending any further surgical intervention.

COMMENT
M. Edward Wilson, MD

I do not think that a hard-and-fast rule on how much hyperopia deserves a trial of spectacles (in presumed infantile esotropia) is needed. I will be quick to try a +2.50 D prescription if the deviation is small and variable, especially if it seems to increase with accommodative effort. On the other hand, I am not likely to try a +2.50-D prescription in an infant with 45Δ of constant esotropia.

As an alternative to glasses, some ophthalmologists have used a trial of topical anticholinesterase inhibitors, such as phospholine iodide 1/8% (limited availability) or di-isofluorophosphate (DFP) (currently not available in the United States), to determine whether there is a refractive element to the esotropia. If a reduction in the esodeviation can be documented, then the glasses will be prescribed.

Surgical Treatment. Surgical realignment of the eyes is the mainstay of ophthalmologic intervention for nonaccommodative early-onset esotropia. The timing of the surgery is affected by the individual patient's medical problems and the variability of the deviation. Because strabismus tends to increase with time in the first year of life, the surgeon should perform at least one examination close to the time of surgery to be certain of the magnitude of the deviation for which graded recession surgery will be performed.

Realignment at younger ages is associated with better outcomes when measured in terms of stability of peripheral binocular function. This fact has led most ophthalmic surgeons in North America to consider the initial corrective surgery for these patients soon after 6 months of age. The completion of the surgical correction within the first 18 months of life should be the goal.

During the past decade, it has been suggested that very early surgery, at 3 to 5 months of age, should be considered when managing infantile esotropia. The presumption is that there is a better chance of establishing binocularity, because less time for anomalous binocular development has been allowed to elapse. Small studies to date have provided conflicting outcome data. One report described several patients with high-grade stereopsis, while a small study of 10 patients found no long-term difference compared with conventionally timed surgery. The Congenital Esotropia Observational Study (CEOS), completed by the Pediatric Eye Disease Investigator Group (PEDIG), found that 27% of esodeviations professionally documented to be greater than 20Δ in the first 4 months of life disappear by 7 months of age. This is particularly true for intermittent deviations and for deviations with angles less than 30Δ. However, even strabismic deviations of 45Δ at 3 months of age resolved without treatment in a number of patients. Given the chance of spontaneous improvement and the modest evidence for benefit, it is premature to recommend very early surgery to correct infantile esotropia.

Most surgeons prefer to perform symmetric surgery for infantile esotropia unless there is significant amblyopia or an anatomic defect in one eye. The surgical dosage is a graded recession of the medial rectus muscles based on the size of the angle (Table 1–1). The strabismic angle for infants is measured at near fixation, using corneal light-reflex testing or prism and alternate cover testing through any prescribed glasses. After the first birthday, an accurate assessment can often be made at distance fixation, eliminating any accommodative component from the measured deviation.

Recession amounts of 3.0 to 6.5 mm from the original insertion have proved quite satisfactory in long-term clinical studies, except for angles exceeding 65Δ. The use of 7.0 mm recessions was proposed for these larger deviations, but these have been reported to have a high rate of consecutive exotropia when performed in the small eyes of infants. This may be due to the retroequatorial placement of the muscle. Large strabismic angles greater than 75Δ, although unusual, have been difficult to manage successfully because of undercorrections frequently encountered with two-muscle surgery. Currently, there is no consensus about whether a patient should have a two-muscle operation (bilateral medial rectus muscle reces-

Table 1–1 Surgical Amount for Esotropia

	Symmetric Surgery	*Unilateral Surgery*	
Deviation (Δ)	*Recession* MR OU (*mm*)	*Recession* MR (*mm*)	*Resection* LR (*mm*)
12–15	3.0	3.0	4.0
16–20	3.5	3.5	5.0
21–25	4.0	4.0	6.0
26–30	4.5	4.5	7.0
31–35	5.0	5.0	8.0
36–40	5.5	5.5	8.5
41–50	6.0	6.0	9.0
>50	6.5		
>70	5.5 + unilateral resection LR 8.0		

LR = lateral rectus; MR = medial rectus; OU = both eyes (*oculi uterque*).

sions) or a three- or four-muscle operation (combining bilateral medial rectus recessions with lateral rectus muscle resections). No randomized, controlled trials have been undertaken to answer this question. For angles of over 75Δ, this author's preference is three-muscle surgery, but reducing the medial rectus muscle recession surgery to 5.5 mm.

COMMENT
M. Edward Wilson, MD

Many surgeons include 7.0 mm in their surgical charts and have not found a larger incidence of late consecutive exotropia compared to 6.0- or 6.5-mm recessions.

COMMENT
Edward G. Buckley, MD

In my experience, the maximum recession of the medial rectus muscle is approximately 12.0 mm from the limbus. Recessions beyond that point tend to result over time in adduction weakness and eventual exotropia. These patients can look good for many years before developing this consecutive exotropia. In all circumstances, there is a duction weakness of the medial rectus that develops over time. For this reason, for deviations larger than 50 D, I perform three-muscle surgery. Attempts to correct deviations greater than 50 D with bilateral medial rectus recessions, in my hands, invariably result in undercorrection.

The target postoperative alignment should be between orthotropia and 8Δ of esodeviation. Exotropic deviations are generally unstable and increase over time. Undercorrections of more than 12Δ should be considered for reoperation.

The management of residual esotropia is individualized. The surgery done most often has been lateral rectus muscle resection of one or both eyes. The author has generally been displeased with the results of this operation, reserving it for patients with prior bilateral medial rectus muscle recessions greater than 5.5 mm. The author's preferred approach for small residual deviations of less than 25Δ is to perform a small re-recession of a single medial rectus muscle if the initial recession was 5.0 mm or less. If the deviation is greater, an ipsilateral small lateral rectus muscle resection is added. This is a powerful surgery, with a risk of a secondary exotropia. When doing the reoperation recess-resect, the author prefers an adjustable-suture technique, briefly waking the child in the postanesthesia care unit, assessing the alignment, and then having additional parenteral sedation administered to allow needed adjustment of the alignment and tying of the sutures.

COMMENT
M. Edward Wilson, MD

There is another reason why medial rectus muscle re-recessions may be better than lateral rectus muscle resections for residual infantile esotropia. When the dissociated strabismus complex is present (any component of it), lateral rectus muscle resections can accentuate dissociated horizontal deviation and lead to more marked manifest dissociated horizontal deviation even when the residual esotropia is well treated. In my opinion, medial rectus muscle re-recessions do not seem to increase the manifest dissociated horizontal deviation as much.

COMMENT
Edward G. Buckley, MD

Since I rarely recess a medial rectus less than 5.0 mm, a re-recession runs the risk of a duction deficit later on. My recommendation is to perform lateral rectus resections, as opposed to trying to re-recess the medial rectus. I agree with Dr. Repka that a resection of the lateral rectus in this situation is extremely powerful, and smaller resections than one would normally perform as an initial procedure should be considered. Thus, 4 or 5 mm resections are quite adequate to correct a fairly large (15 to 25 D) residual deviation. I rarely perform bilateral lateral rectus resections for this reason. Like overrecessed medial rectus muscles, bilaterally resected lateral rectus muscles will initially look good, but over time an exodeviation can result. This consecutive exodeviation is more likely to occur the farther back the medial rectus muscles were recessed as an initial procedure.

Differential Diagnosis. The differential diagnosis of early-onset esotropia, besides early-onset refractive esotropia, includes Duane syndrome, abducens nerve palsy/paresis, nystagmus blockage syndrome, sensory esotropia, and Möbius syndrome.

Duane syndrome. The Duane syndrome presents very early in childhood as an esotropia, a head turn, or unusual eye movements. The entity, a form of ocular motor aberrant innervation, appears to be due to a loss of appropriate innervation of the affected muscle. Clinically, this occurs most often when there is a deficiency of the sixth (abducens) nerve innervation to the lateral rectus muscle, resulting in a weakness of ipsilateral abduction. Electromyogram recordings have found no enhancement of lateral rectus muscle activity on attempted *ab*duction but paradoxical muscle activity in the lateral rectus on attempted *ad*duction. In one case, the abducens nerve was absent on the affected side, and innervation came from branches of the third (oculomotor) nerve. The affected muscle generally shows discrete areas of fibrosis and normal muscle fibers, the latter where there is innervation.

The most common form of Duane syndrome has limited abduction and a small esotropia. It is termed *type I* or *esotropic Duane syndrome*. The key findings include the relatively small esodeviation in primary position, lateral-gaze incomitance, and eyelid fissure changes with horizontal-gaze shifts, which are not seen with other forms of esotropia. The small primary-position deviation is out of proportion to the usually marked abduction deficiency. A widening of the fissure on attempted abduction and a narrowing of the fissure on adduction characterize the eyelid fissure changes. These are not always apparent in young children.

Sixth nerve palsy. Abducens (sixth) nerve paresis/palsy is uncommon in children. It is common for children with infantile esotropia to have apparent abduction weakness on voluntary ductions. Inspection of eye movements on oculocephalic testing (doll's-head maneuver) will often help make this distinction, demonstrating near-normal abduction with good velocity in infantile esotropia.

Nystagmus blockage syndrome. The nystagmus blockage syndrome (NBS) is a type of early-onset esotropia. It should be considered in patients with varying esotropic deviations and nystagmus. The syndrome is defined by von Noorden as characterizing a patient with early-onset variable esotropia who is orthotropic with manifest nystagmus when inattentive and esotropic with minimal nystagmus when attentive. The patient likely becomes esotropic because of sustained convergence. Specific attention during the examination to pupillary constriction during the esotropic phase may help to establish the diagnosis. The treatment of this condition includes large medial rectus muscle recessions, so that from a therapeutic aspect, there is not much difference between the management of this condition and that of other forms of esotropia. Recurrence of the esotropia is higher with NBS than with other forms of esotropia.

COMMENT
Edward G. Buckley, MD

My experience with NBS is that fairly typical amounts of medial rectus muscle recession are all that is necessary. I have been surprised when several patients who had medial rectus recessions for this syndrome became relatively straight for a while and then developed a head turn. This certainly complicates subsequent nystagmus surgery.

COMMENT
David A. Plager, MD

Our experience with this entity has included a significantly higher rate of recurrent esotropia when conventional amounts of medial rectus recession are used. These patients tend to "eat up" surgery designed to lessen the esotropia, whether medial rectus recession or later lateral rectus resection.

Sensory esotropia. Disruption of visual input in childhood often produces an ocular misalignment, which is most often an esotropia. Therefore, all children with esotropia should be examined to exclude a problem with the afferent visual pathway.

Möbius syndrome. The Möbius syndrome is caused by a malformation of the brain stem, producing hypoplasia of one or more cranial nerves. Involvement of the abducens nerve leads to the esotropia. Other cranial nerve dysfunction can lead to difficulties with feeding and breathing and to corneal hypesthesia. Skeletal and limb malformations may be present.

ACQUIRED ESOTROPIA

Acquired esotropia is a nonspecific term for a heterogeneous collection of strabismic cases. The only common feature is the onset of the deviation after 6 months of age. These conditions include refractive esotropia, accommodative refractive esotropia, basic nonrefractive esotropia, and a number of neuro-ophthalmologic conditions leading to crossing of the eyes.

Refractive Esotropia. The most common form of acquired esotropia is refractive esotropia. This condition, often familial, usually begins in the first 3 years of life but can occur up to 6 or 7 years of age. The patient commonly presents with insidious, intermittent, and increasing amounts of crossing. Other symptoms include squinting of the eyelids or covering an eye, presumably to eliminate the diplopia. Acquired esotropia is associated with high amounts of hypermetropia, generally +3.00 D or more. Usually no inferior oblique muscle overaction, dissociated strabismus complex, or latent nystagmus is associated with this form of esotropia, although the presence of these conditions does not exclude the diagnosis. Patients with acquired esotropia should undergo a thorough ophthalmologic examination, with emphasis on cycloplegic retinoscopy. Examination of the optic nerves should specifically evaluate the patient for papilledema in every case of recently acquired esotropia to exclude increased intracranial pressure.

Patients with acquired esotropic deviations and significant hyperopia should be placed in the full hypermetropic correction as determined by a cycloplegic refraction. These glasses are usually well tolerated even in school-age children. However, if the child is having difficulty adapting to the glasses, a trial of 1 or more weeks of daily topical atropine solution 1% is prescribed. Atropine eliminates any residual accommodation, which may otherwise cause blurred vision, making the glasses acceptable to the child. For patients with small-angle, intermittent esotropia, an initial trial of partial hypermetropic correction is reasonable, but the family needs to understand that the lenses may need to be replaced with those providing full hypermetropic correction if the partial correction does not control the deviation.

The patient should wear the glasses full-time for at least 4 weeks. This will ensure that the patient has had ample time to relax the accommodative tone before returning for a visit to see whether the glasses are successful. The glasses are considered successful only if the strabismic angle is reduced to less than 10Δ, ideally to orthotropia. If glasses do not reduce the deviation to less than 10Δ, another cycloplegic refraction should be performed. Additional hypermetropic refractive error may be discovered at this refraction. If this is found, the spectacle power should be increased and the glasses worn for another 4-week period.

Children successfully treated with glasses or contact lenses will continue to wear them for the next few years. Over time, many patients experience a reduction in either their hypermetropia or their accommodative convergence. Each of these changes will allow the power of the glasses to be reduced—in some cases, even removed.

Some surgeons, especially outside North America, have suggested that patients with refractive esotropia responsive to glasses could be managed with surgery and never with lenses. However, the children are subjected to surgery that may not be necessary, as they may become less hypermetropic and not esotropic as they grow older. There are additional drawbacks for children with higher hypermetropia. Surgery makes these patients exotropic, inducing an accommodative vergence to return the eyes to a straight alignment. Often, this vergence cannot be sustained over time, and the surgically created exotropic deviation may become manifest. Furthermore, these children cannot sustain the needed accommodative effort for sharp vision. Glasses must be prescribed, producing clear vision but also exotropia. The author therefore does not recommend this approach.

If a residual esodeviation remains despite full cycloplegic correction, the patient is a candidate for strabismus surgery. The typical angles vary from 12 to 45Δ. Generally, bilateral medial rectus muscle recessions of a graduated amount are performed for the deviation measured through the glasses at distance fixation. Undercorrection is common with the surgical management of this condition. To reduce the frequency of undercorrection, some surgeons operate for the near angle, an average of near and distance, or use a table with augmented surgical dosages.

A randomized clinical trial funded by the National Eye Institute has found that the use of preoperative prism adaptation can modestly increase the chance of obtaining successful realignment in this patient population. The study found that the motor success rate was improved from 79% to 89% when surgery for the prism-adapted angle was performed. This technique involves placing Fresnel prisms over the patient's spectacles to neutralize the distance strabismic angle. The patient is then measured weekly or biweekly to detect a "buildup" in the angle and to increase the prisms to account for that angle. If the patient has a fusion response and the prism-adapted angle is stable (that is, not increasing further), the patient should have surgery for the built-up angle. This approach reduces the frequency of undercorrection. The chance of overcorrection, even with prism-adapted surgery, is quite low. High-grade stereopsis is restored in about 50% of the patients.

Postoperative undercorrected patients should remain in full hypermetropic correction. If there is residual esotropia of greater than 12Δ, additional surgery should be considered on the lateral rectus muscles or on one of the recessed medial rectus muscles. Postoperative overcorrected patients may have a reduction of the plus sphere to manipulate the residual deviation by stimulating accommodative convergence. This may allow a temporary "cure" of the strabismus, though ultimately further surgery may be necessary.

Accommodative Non-Refractive Esotropia. Accommodative non-refractive esotropia, also termed *high accommodative convergence/accommodation ratio* (AC/A), is an acquired esodeviation in which the near angle is greater than the distance angle by more than 10Δ (clinical definition). These patients have either no deviation or a small esotropia at distance, a small amount of hypermetropic error, and a large near angle. They typically range from 2 to 6 years of age at diagnosis. There is usually no inferior oblique muscle overaction, latent nystagmus, or dissociated strabismus complex. A complete ophthalmologic examination, including cycloplegic retinoscopy, is necessary. These children typically present with intermittent crossing, generally at near fixation, which often results in a delay in detection of 6 months or more. The most common treatment is a full cycloplegic correction for distance. A bifocal add of +2.50 or +3.00 D is prescribed for children with good distance alignment but more than 10Δ of esotropia at near fixation. Many children adapt to this treatment very well, with good fusion at near and distance fixation. As they progress toward the teenage years, progressive or blended bifocals can be used.

COMMENT

Gunter K. von Noorden, MD

I am having difficulty with the term *accomodative refractive esotropia* for an esotropia that is greater at near than at distance fixation because of a high AC/A ratio. This term implies that the refractive error plays a role in the etiology. However, this is not the case. A high AC/A ratio is independent of the underlying refractive error and may be found in hypermetropic, emmetropic, or myopic patients. We prefer the term *non-refractive accommodative esotropia* for this condition to distinguish it clearly from *refractive acccomodative esotropia*, in which esotropia is caused by excessive accomodative convergence elicited by an uncovered hypermetropic refractive error.

Bifocals should not be considered permanent. These patients should be examined to confirm that wearing the lens decreases the near angle to the monofixation range (less than 10Δ). Sensory evidence of binocular function should be sought. Other clues to a functional benefit may be the voluntary use of the bifocal segment, evident in preverbal children by a chin-up posture for near activities. Bifocals may be useful during the treatment of amblyopia, as many such patients have decreased accommodative facility. However, if the angle is not sufficiently reduced to allow an improvement in fusion, the bifocals may be discontinued.

Bifocal usage should be reassessed as these patients grow older and sensory function can be adequately assessed. Binocular function, such as stereopsis, measured at near fixation through the add should be better than that measured at near fixation through the distance segment. The documentation of a benefit is sufficient to continue their use. Many teenagers prefer contact lenses, so the nearly universal question seems to be "For how long should bifocals be prescribed?" The basic rule is that bifocals should be maintained only as long they reduce the deviation of the eyes to less than 10Δ and produce some element of sensory fusion. If these benefits are not evident, then the bifocals may be as much an aesthetic blemish as the in-turning deviation. One solution is the use of progressive or blended bifocals, which can be worn very successfully by children and adolescents. However, this cannot solve the "problem" of the glasses.

The successful bifocal wearer often experiences a spontaneous reduction in the AC/A ratio between 10 and 15 years of age. This will allow reduction in the power of the bifocal add. Weaning by 0.75 to 1.00 D each year is often a successful strategy. For those patients who cannot be weaned, surgery may be considered to dispense with the bifocal lenses. Such surgery is most successful in patients with sensory fusion. The surgical dose may be based on the mean of the distance and near angles measured through the distance lens. Some clinicians have reported good results using prism adaptation for this situation. They prescribe distance lenses with Fresnel press-on prisms neutralizing the near angle over the entire lens. With this approach, if the patient does not become exotropic at distance, surgery for the angle based on the size of the prism correction is indicated.

Patients who do not demonstrate sufficient realignment of the eyes at distance or at near fixation despite hypermetropic correction with bifocals should be considered for surgery. Without such correction, there is little chance of their eventually developing binocular vision.

Surgery performed for the distance angle is insufficient to realign the eyes when a high AC/A ratio is present. Some surgeons operate for the near angle, others for the average of the near and distant angles measured through the distance correction. Such surgery should consist of bilateral medial rectus recession, which seems to enhance the surgical impact at near fixation. This may also be a situation where a combined recession and posterior fixation suture may be helpful. The use of preoperative prism adaptation for the near angle has been suggested but remains unproven.

COMMENT

Edward G. Buckley, MD

I have found that bilateral medial rectus fadenoperations can be quite effective in dealing with high AC/A ratio esotropia, which cannot be treated effectively by bifocals. In this circumstance, large bilateral medial rectus recessions usually result in a subsequent exotropia with time. Bilateral medial rectus fadenoperations allow the distance deviation to remain stable while reducing the near deviation significantly. This approach can also be considered for individuals who cannot be weaned from bifocal glasses over time. I usually reserve this approach for those individuals who have had bifocal correction, relatively good stability of the angle, and some binocular function, and who reach the early teen years and want to wear contact lenses.

In this circumstance, it is reasonable to consider a surgical approach, and I have found the bilateral medial rectus fadenoperation to be very successful.

Acquired Non-refractive Esotropia. Acquired non-refractive esotropia presents after 6 months of age with minimal hypermetropia or no response to hypermetropic spectacles. Once a cycloplegic refraction has shown insignificant hypermetropia and an examination has ruled out other disease conditions and confirmed complete abduction, the child should undergo bilateral medial rectus muscle recession for the amount of the deviation. These patients may also benefit from prism-adaptation techniques if the esodeviation is small.

Acute Comitant Esotropia. Although most forms of acquired esotropia are comitant, the term *acute comitant esotropia* is reserved for a particular form of apparently acute acquired esotropia. Usually over the age of 5 years, these patients suddenly develop a comitant esotropia without evidence of abduction weakness. A few have substantial hypermetropia and probably represent late-onset refractive esotropia. Another small number experience onset of the esodeviation following trauma or illness. However, this clinical profile is important to recognize because it may also occur in the setting of intracranial disease, such as hydrocephalus, pseudotumor cerebri, Chiari malformation, or even neoplasia, usually tumors of the posterior fossa. Therefore, patients over the age of 5 years with new esotropia and without significant hypermetropic error should have a careful examination of the optic disc and some form of neuroimaging. If the results of the fundus examination and scan are normal and the esotropic deviation is stable, the patient may undergo bilateral medial rectus muscle recession to correct the deviation. Restoration of high-grade stereopsis is common when the duration of strabismus is short and the condition is not associated with neoplasia.

Divergence Paralysis or Insufficiency. An esotropia worse at distance than at near, when measured with full cycloplegic correction and full ocular ductions, may be defined as *divergence insufficiency* (chronic symptoms) or *paralysis* (acute onset). This condition may represent mild abduction deficits that cannot be detected with the examination of the ocular ductions. However, in some cases, slowed abducting saccades can be elicited. The acute-onset form can be associated with brain stem disease, particularly demyelination, or neuromuscular disease. Neuroimaging is indicated, although in most cases the results will be normal. Neurologic consultation should be obtained if there are other symptoms. Some patients with divergence paralysis recover completely, although recovery can take up to 1 year. Symptomatic relief can be provided with prism—in many cases, a Fresnel prism over the distance segment of the glasses.

Long-standing deviations are managed with muscle surgery. If there is no ductional deficit, both medial rectus muscles are recessed. If there is evidence of weakness of a lateral rectus muscle, then a resection of that lateral rectus muscle and a recession of the ipsilateral medial rectus muscle may be preferred.

COMMENT

Gunter K. von Noorden, MD

The differential diagnosis between divergence paralysis and bilateral sixth nerve paresis may be difficult. In both instances, the esotropia is limited to distance fixation. However, mild abduction deficits and decreased saccadic velocity are features of bilateral sixth nerve paresis, not of a defective divergence mechanism. Another distinguishing feature of bilateral sixth nerve paresis is a subtle increase in esotropia when measured in maximal lateral versions as compared to the primary position.

COMMENT

Marshall M. Parks, MD

This chapter clearly illustrates the difference between early-onset esotropia (prior to the development of binocular vision reflexes) and later-onset esotropia (after the development of binocular vision reflexes). The differences are in both the sensory and motor areas. In the sensory area, the big difference is between early-onset infantile esotropes, who have inherited the genetically determined inability to develop macular binocular vision, and late-onset esotropes, who present after their binocular reflexes have developed. The latter group develop both macular and extramacular binocular vision reflexes. Early-onset esotropia patients develop only the extramacular binocular vision reflexes and only if their alignment has been surgically accomplished by approximately 2 years of age. Macular binocular vision is a fragile reflex compared to the durable extramacular binocular vision reflex. Macular binocular vision requires constant reinforcement to survive; 3 months of constant absence of reinforcement destroys the reflex, which appears not to be age-related.

Loss of macular binocular vision function is characterized by replacement of bifixation with monofixation and a 3° macular scotoma appearing in the nonfixating eye, replacement of previously excellent stereoacuity by poor stereoacuity, and amblyopia appearing in children unless they alternate their fixation. This chain of events carries a very sobering message to caregivers. To avoid permanent loss of macular binocular vision, appropriate care must be delivered promptly. Ideally, it should be instituted during the intermittent phase of the esotropia that characterizes its onset. The fault for the delay lies among the triad of parents, primary care physician, and ophthalmologist. All need to become better educated about the urgent need to deliver prompt care to the child who is just beginning to manifest intermittent esotropia.

Suggested Readings

Helveston EM, Neely DF, Stidham DB, et al: Results of early alignment of congenital esotropia. *Ophthalmology* 1999; 106:1716–1726.

Pediatric Eye Disease Investigator Group: The clinical spectrum of early-onset esotropia: experience of the Congenital Esotropia Observational Study. *Am J Ophthalmol* 2002; 133:102–108.

Pediatric Eye Disease Investigator Group: Spontaneous resolution of early-onset esotropia: experience of the Congenital Esotropia Observational Study. *Am J Ophthalmol* 2002; 133:109–118.

Prism Adaptation Research Group: Efficacy of prism adaptation in the surgical management of acquired esotropia. *Arch Ophthalmol* 1990; 108:1248–1256.

von Noorden GK: *Binocular Vision and Ocular Motility: Theory and Management of Strabismus*, 5th ed. St Louis: CV Mosby Co; 1996.

Wright KW, Edelman PM, McVey JH, et al: High-grade stereo acuity after early surgery for congenital esotropia. *Arch Ophthalmol* 1994; 112:913–919.

2

Exotropic Deviations

M. EDWARD WILSON

Divergent strabismus is known as *exotropia*. Because the exodeviation may be controlled by fusion mechanisms, it is most accurate to label these deviations *exophoria*, *intermittent exotropia*, or *constant exotropia*, according to whether fusion mechanisms contain the deviation in a latent form for all, part, or none of the waking hours, respectively. Exodeviations are said to occur less frequently than esodeviations. However, many patients with exophoria and well-controlled intermittent exotropia never seek ophthalmologic care and are most likely underrepresented when incidence calculations are based on the frequency of diagnosis in a strabismus practice. While the exact cause of most exodeviations is unknown, proposed causes include anatomic and mechanical factors within the orbit, as well as innervational abnormalities such as excessive tonic divergence. A hereditary basis for exodeviation is apparent in some families.

Exophoria is a type of exodeviation controlled by fusion mechanisms under conditions of normal binocular vision. Exophorias are detected when binocular vision is interrupted, as during an alternate cover test. Constant exotropia, by contrast, is a manifest exodeviation not controlled by fusion mechanisms, so the visual axes are never properly aligned. Constant exotropia may occur over time as fusional control is lost, as in an intermittent exotropia that gradually becomes constant. Another form of constant exotropia, sensory exotropia, can be caused by any condition that reduces visual acuity in one eye. While children younger than 5 years of age commonly develop esotropia after unilateral visual loss, older children and adults usually develop exotropia.

The most common type of exodeviation seen in an ophthalmologic practice is intermittent exotropia, which is latent at some times and manifest at others. Intermittent exotropia is not only the most common but also the most challenging type of exodeviation to cure long term. Therefore, much of this chapter concerns intermittent exotropia. Less common but nonetheless important exodeviations, such as congenital exotropia, convergence insufficiency, and exotropic Duane syndrome, are also discussed. Dissociated horizontal deviation is covered in Chapter 4, "Dissociated Deviations."

INTERMITTENT EXOTROPIA

Clinical Characteristics. Intermittent exotropia often begins before the age of 5 years, but when it is well controlled, the deviation may be detected for the first time much later in childhood. The frequency of the episodes of manifest exotropia may remain unchanged for many years, even for life. However, as discussed below, progression toward constancy is often seen. Although normal newborns often manifest an exodeviation in the first few months of life (prior to the development of fixation, accommodation, and binocularity), by 6 months of age most infants have well-developed fixation, following movements, and well-aligned eyes. Any infant 6 months of age or older who presents with a large-angle, poorly controlled intermittent exotropia that manifests frequently even at near may rapidly progress to constant exotropia. Early-onset intermittent exotropia (Fig. 2–1) with progression toward constancy must be distinguished from congenital exotropia (discussed later in the chapter), because the prognosis is better and neurologic problems are less commonly associated with the former condition. Most intermittent exotropia, however, is well controlled early in life and presents for treatment later in childhood or even in adulthood (Fig. 2–2).

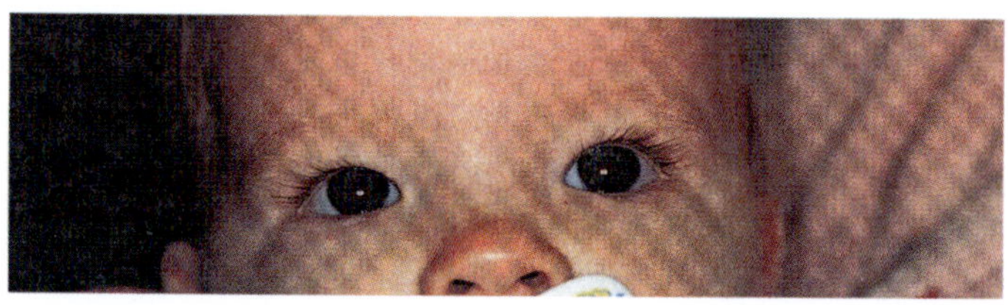

A

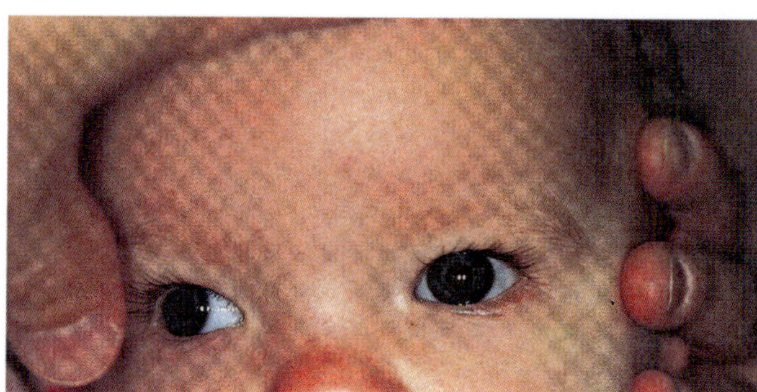

B

Figure 2–1. A 7-month-old infant with early-onset intermittent exotropia. (*A*) Well-aligned eyes. (*B*) Large-angle exotropia. The Examiner's thumb was used as an occluder and has just been removed from in front of the right eye. This large deviation was manifest frequently at near as well as at distance fixation. It progressed over a few months to nearly constant exotropia. Surgery was performed, with a good result. (Part B reprinted with permission from Wilson ME Jr: Exotropia. *Focal Points: Clinical Modules for Ophthalmologists.* San Francisco: American Academy of Ophthalmology; vol 13, no 11, 1995).

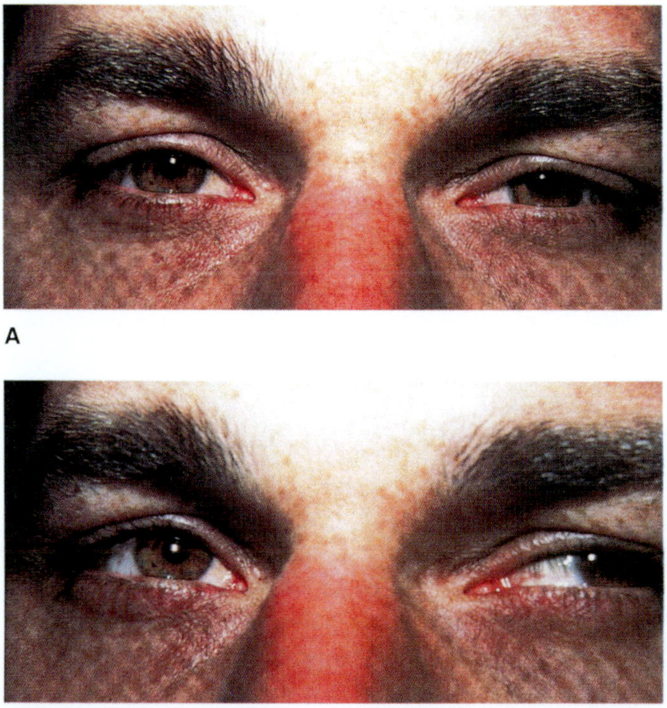

A

B

Figure 2–2. Large-angle intermittent exotropia presenting in adulthood. (*A*) Well-aligned eyes. (*B*) Large-angle exotropia. The deviation was likely present for many years but was well controlled until recently. The patient underwent surgery because exotropia was now becoming manifest more often during the daytime.

COMMENT

Michael X. Repka, MD

The natural history of intermittent exotropia in young childhood and in those of early school age is not well characterized. The exact percentage of patients who actually do progress is unknown. I suspect it is less than the 50% often cited. The impact of nonsurgical treatments compared to observation is also unknown.

Since proper eye alignment in intermittent exotropia requires that compensatory fusional factors be active, the deviation often becomes manifest during times of visual inattention, fatigue, or stress. Parents of affected children often report that exotropia occurs late in the day with fatigue or during illness, daydreaming, drowsiness upon awakening, or when the child is being scolded. Closure of one eye is often seen with exposure to bright light. In childhood, the deviation of the eyes is usually larger for distance viewing than for near. Parents often report that the exodeviation manifests more frequently when the visual target is remote. In adults, near and distant exodeviations tend to be more equal in magnitude, even if fusional control remains good. Intermittent exotropia can be associated with small hypertropias, A and V patterns, and oblique muscle dysfunction. Inferior oblique muscle overaction can be detected in about one-third of patients.

In many but not all patients, untreated intermittent exotropia progresses toward constant exotropia, typically evolving through four phases:

1. Exophoria at distance, orthophoria at near
2. Intermittent exotropia at distance, orthophoria or exophoria at near
3. Exotropia at distance, exophoria or intermittent exotropia at near
4. Exotropia at distance, exotropia at near

COMMENT

Gunter K. von Noorden, MD

The classification of exodeviation into four groups according to differences of the deviation at near and distance fixation was in vogue long before introduction of the occlusion test by Scobee and Burian and before Brown measured the near deviation through +3.00 D spherical lenses. In fact, this classification was proposed by Alexander Duane as early as 1897. It remains useful in a descriptive sense to distinguish between exodeviations with different near/distance characteristics, but it must be recognized that this terminology has no etiologic implications. There is no evidence to suggest that a *divergence excess* or *convergence insufficiency* exodeviation is caused by an actual excess of divergence innervation in the former or insufficiency of convergence in the latter. We have suggested speaking of a divergence excess *type* or convergence insufficiency *type* of exodeviation when using these terms.

As exotropia progresses, tropic episodes occur with less fatigue and last longer than previously. Initial diplopia during manifest exotropia is rapidly replaced by the cortical adaptations of suppression and abnormal retinal correspondence. Bifixation and high-grade stereopsis can be maintained when the eyes are well aligned, even as suppression and abnormal retinal correspondence develop to rid the patient of diplopia and visual confusion when the eyes are deviated. Amblyopia is uncommon in intermittent exotropia unless progression to constant or nearly constant exotropia occurs in early childhood.

Clinical Evaluation. The clinical evaluation begins with a detailed history to determine as accurately as possible the age of onset of the strabismus and whether the exotropia is progressing toward constancy. The examiner should record how often and under what specific circumstances the manifest exotropia occurs. Whether recovery to straight eyes occurs rapidly should also be recorded. Often, the intermittent exotropia will begin to manifest more frequently (with less and less fatigue) and simultaneously for longer periods of time before recovery to straight eyes. Control of the exodeviation exhibited throughout the examination can be categorized as good, fair, or poor (Fig. 2–3):

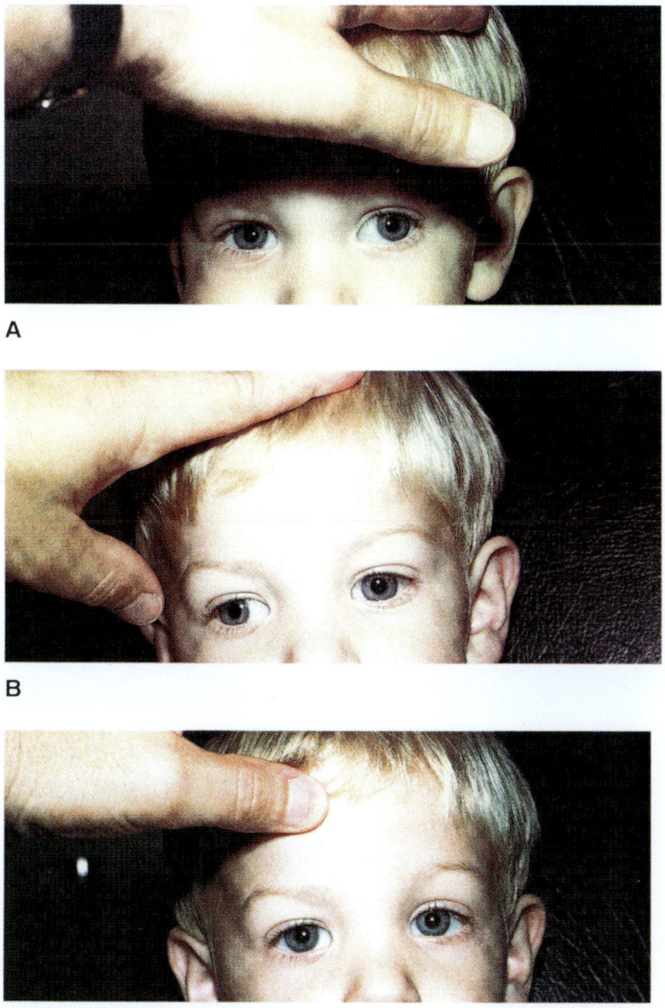

A

B

C

Figure 2–3. A 3-year-old boy with intermittent exotropia. Fair office control was demonstrated. Exotropia became manifest after fusion was disrupted by cover testing. Fusion resumed only after a few blinks. (*A*) Exodeviation of the left eye. (*B*) Exodeviation of the right eye. (C) Recovery to straight eyes after alternate cover testing was complete.

1. *Good office control:* exotropia is manifest only after cover testing; fusion resumes rapidly, without blinking or refixating.
2. *Fair office control:* exotropia is manifest after fusion is disrupted by cover testing; fixation resumes only after blinking or refixating.
3. *Poor office control:* exotropia is manifest spontaneously in the office without disruption of fusion.

Strabismus measurements are best taken in the primary (straight-ahead) position at 20 ft (6 m) and at 14 in., using a target that controls accommodation. A light source should never be used as a fixation target when measuring an exodeviation, because it does not prevent overaccommodation, which will reduce the deviation. In very young patients, in whom corneal light-reflection measurements must be used, a detailed picture or toy should be placed over or beside the light to control accommodation. To bring out the maximum exodeviation, two additional measurements, an outdoor measurement and a postocclusion measurement, are important.

For a proper outdoor measurement, the patient should view through a window a far distant target (such as a flagpole on a building a quarter of a mile away). Because both increased illumination and the distance of the target from the patient may be important to finding the maximum deviation, the patient should stand as close to the window as possible while still allowing the examiner to stand between the patient and the window to obtain the strabismus measurements. For the postocclusion measurement, 60 minutes of monocular occlusion is recommended, although 30 minutes is commonly used and is probably more practical for the office setting. The postocclusion measurement is performed at 20 ft.

Measurements in right and left gaze should also be taken, since many surgeons recommend reducing the amount of surgery if the exodeviation measures significantly less in side gaze than in primary gaze. When an American-made plastic prism is used for side-gaze measurements, it is best to hold the prism over the adducted eye with the posterior face of the prism perpendicular to the line of sight. Improper prism positioning can simulate lateral-gaze incomitance. Small reductions in side-gaze measurement, as compared to the primary position, should be ignored. This author defines *significant* lateral-gaze incomitance as a reduction in side gaze of 50% or more compared to the primary position.

Intermittent exotropia has traditionally been classified into four groups, based on the difference between alternating prism and cover measurements at distance and near and the change in the near measurement produced by prolonged unilateral occlusion or +3.00 diopter (D) lenses (Table 2–1). It must be noted that +3.00 D lenses relax accommodative as well as fusional convergence and therefore may be less useful for classification compared to prolonged occlusion. This classification is still used by some surgeons for surgical planning.

COMMENT

Gunter K. von Noorden, MD

The results of the occlusion test must be kept apart from the effect of +3.00 lenses at near fixation: +3.00 spherical lenses eliminate the need to accommodate at a fixation distance of 33 cm. I am unaware of such lenses also having an effect on fusional convergence, as stated in this chapter. This in-

Table 2–1 Classification of Intermittent Exotropia

Type	*Examination Measurement Parameters*
Basic	Distance and near are equal
Divergence excess	Distance exceeds near by ≥15Δ
Convergence insufficiency	Near exceeds distance by ≥15Δ
Simulated (or pseudo-) divergence excess	Distance initially exceeds near, but near equals distance after 30 to 60 minutes of uniocular occlusion

crease of exophoria when accommodation is suspended must be considered a normal and predictable response in a patient with a high accommodative convergence/accommodation ratio (AC/A), not a manifestation of a hidden exodeviation. Why then do the +3.00 spherical lens test at all? As Brown pointed out, a good reason for knowing the AC/A ratio prior to surgery is to identify those patients who may benefit from prescription of even a mild hypermetropic refractive error or from miotics in case of overcorrection.

Recently, it has been recognized that differences between distance and near measurements in intermittent exotropia are most likely not due to divergence or convergence abnormalities. Rather, fusional aftereffects, known as *tenacious proximal fusion*, are to blame. Furthermore, the gradient AC/A ratio in most of these patients is normal after these fusional aftereffects are suspended by prolonged unilateral occlusion. A measurement of the deviation at 14 in. and at 20 ft after 60 minutes of unilateral occlusion is recommended. Measurement of the gradient AC/A ratio at distance using −2.00 D lenses is also recommended to detect the rare patient with a true high AC/A ratio. This AC/A ratio measurement must occur after fusional aftereffects are suspended by unilateral occlusion.

COMMENT

Edward G. Buckley, MD

Determining the full amount of exotropia present is often challenging. In children, distance fixation is often difficult to achieve with any reliability, and the near deviation is often nonexistent or markedly less. Using a +3.00 lens to relax accommodation in most circumstances gives the same exodeviation present at distance after occlusion. While acknowledging that tenacious proximal fusion and high AC/A ratios may play a role, if the +3.00 measurement at near is within 5 prism diopters (Δ) of the distance measurement, I routinely operate for this amount.

An *ultranear* measurement can be substituted for the gradient AC/A ratio calculation. After unilateral occlusion, a measurement is taken at 7 in. (half the standard 14-in. distance). Patients with a true high AC/A ratio will likely demonstrate an esodeviation when measured at ultranear. Intermittent exotropia patients with a normal AC/A ratio will not demonstrate an esodeviation, regardless of how close the target is held to the eyes. This author has found the ultranear measurement after occlusion to be a quick and reliable screening test for those rare patients with a true high AC/A ratio. A formal measurement of the gradient AC/A ratio is then unnecessary. Patients with a true high AC/A ratio are often treated differently than patients with a normal AC/A ratio, as discussed in the section "Surgical Treatment."

Sensory testing usually reveals excellent stereopsis with normal retinal correspondence when the exodeviation is latent and suppression with abnormal retinal correspondence when the exotropia is manifest. However, if the deviation manifests very rarely, diplopia may persist during manifest exotropia. Some find it useful to measure stereopsis at 20 ft as well as at 14 in., because reduced distance stereopsis may indicate poor control of the distance exodeviation.

Nonsurgical Treatment. Corrective lenses are prescribed for significant myopic, astigmatic, and hyperopic refractive errors. Myopic correction, even if mild, may improve control of the exodeviation. In addition to having retinal blur for distance viewing, uncorrected myopes have reduced accommodative demand and thus reduced accommodative convergence, which may lessen control of the exodeviation. Mild to moderate degrees of hyperopia are not routinely corrected in children with intermittent exotropia for fear of worsening the deviation. However, some patients with more than 4.00 D of hyperopia (or more than 1.50 D of hyperopic anisometropia) may actually have better control of the exodeviation after optical correction. Children with severe hyperopia may be unable to sustain the necessary accommodation for a clear image. The lack of accommodative effort produces a blurred retinal image and manifest exotropia. Optical correction may improve retinal image clarity and help control the exodeviation.

Additional minus lens power, usually 2.00 to 4.00 D beyond refractive error correction, is used by some physicians to temporarily stimulate accommodative convergence and help control the exodeviation. This therapy may be very effective as a temporizing measure to promote fusion and avoid surgery during the most visually immature years, when amblyopia and loss of stereopsis can occur after a surgical overcorrection. One study found no increase in myopia or myopic progression in children using minus lens therapy compared to controls. However, these lenses may cause asthenopia in older children.

A rare but distinct group of intermittent exotropia patients have a true high AC/A ratio when measured after fusional aftereffects have been eliminated by 30 to 60 minutes of unilateral patching. With conventional surgery, these patients often overcorrect to a high AC/A ratio accommodative esotropia. Minus lenses and bifocals may effectively control the deviation in this small group of patients without the need for surgery.

Small to moderate deviations sometimes can be treated effectively with alternate part-time patching (or patching of the dominant, nondeviating eye) for 5 to 6 hours per day. The benefit, however, is often temporary. The exact mechanism by which patching improves control of intermittent exotropia is not known. Presumably, patching disrupts suppression in some manner and is characterized as a passive orthoptic treatment.

Active orthoptic treatments, consisting of antisuppression therapy with diplopia awareness and fusional convergence training, can be used alone or in combination with patching, minus lenses, or surgery. Although very successful with some patients, usually those with less than 30Δ of deviation, the home and office treatment protocols that have been studied have received mixed reviews. Fusional convergence training works best for patients with a remote near point of convergence or poor fusional amplitudes. Antisuppression therapy and diplopia awareness training provide the patient with a sensory biofeedback mechanism (diplopia) that stimulates the fusional vergence system. For deviations of 20Δ or less, orthoptic treatment has been reported by some to have a long-term success rate comparable to that of surgery. Others have found no benefit and recommend surgery for any deviation that is poorly controlled.

In patients old enough to cooperate, fusional convergence training should be considered for those with intermittent exotropia and reduced fusional convergence amplitudes or a remote near point of convergence. Although more controversial, antisuppression therapy with diplopia awareness training may be appropriate when suppression is dense, especially when the deviation is 25 to 30Δ or less and the patient is old enough to cooperate with treatment (6 to 7 years of age). In general, an active orthoptic program for intermittent exotropia would combine fusional vergence training and antisuppression therapy. Patients often require 10 to 20 office visits. Training is begun at near (where the patient has the best fusion) and progresses to intermediate and then far distances. An attempt is made to eliminate suppression. Theoretically, eliminating suppression can lead to constant diplopia if fusion is not present. This risk is more real with constant deviations, especially esotropia, and less so with intermittent exotropia.

Many therapists recommend training mostly *in free space*, rather than *in instrument*. Divergence training is often done, as well as convergence training. Because data on the effectiveness of this latter orthoptic treatment conflict, further study is needed to define patients who might benefit. In addition, the preoperative and postoperative roles of orthoptic treatment remain unclear.

Base-in prisms can be used to promote fusion in intermittent exotropia, but this treatment option is seldom chosen for long-term management because it is likely to reduce fusional vergence amplitudes.

Surgical Treatment. Many patients with intermittent exotropia ultimately require surgery, customarily performed when progression toward constant exotropia is documented despite the use of appropriate nonsurgical treatments. However, consensus is lacking regarding specific indications. Some surgeons advocate very early surgery for any deviation of 15Δ or more that is manifest daily. The purpose is to realign the eyes before suppression becomes firmly established and to stabilize proper alignment over the long term. Other surgeons reserve surgery for patients who have progressed to nearly constant exotropia and often advise withholding surgery whenever possible in very young patients to avoid amblyopia and loss of fine stereopsis, which could result from an overcorrection with constant esodeviation. Close postoperative follow-up, however, minimizes these risks.

Some surgeons perform unilateral recess-resect (medial rectus muscle resection combined with lateral rectus muscle recession) for patients in the basic and simulated divergence excess categories; bilateral lateral rectus muscle recession for those with true divergence excess; and bilateral medial rectus muscle resection for those with the convergence insufficiency type of intermittent exotropia. This surgical scheme was based on the belief that medial rectus muscle surgery had more effect at near and that lateral rectus muscle surgery had more effect at distance. Simulated divergence excess patients were treated similarly to the basic type of exotropia because it was believed that these patients actually had a near deviation that equaled the distance deviation, but that it was masked by fusional vergences at near.

Recent studies have placed in doubt the belief that medial rectus muscle surgery has more effect at near and lateral rectus muscle surgery has more effect at dis-

Table 2–2 Surgical Amount for Exotropia*

Deviation (Δ)	*Recession* LR OU (*mm*)	*Resection* MR OU (*mm*)
15	4.0	3.0
20	5.0	4.0
25	6.0	5.0
30	7.0	5.5
35	7.5	6.0
40	8.0+	6.5
50	9.0+	7.0

LR = lateral rectus; MR = medial rectus; OU = both eyes (*oculi uterque*)

*These surgical numbers are only a guide and must be modified by the surgeon's own experience. The surgical amount for symmetric bilateral surgery is given in the second and third columns. For unilateral recess-resect procedures, the number in each column is used for a given deviation. Surgery on three horizontal muscles is often selected for deviations above 50Δ. The author prefers to recess both lateral rectus muscles 8.0 mm and add a graded medial rectus muscle resection as the third muscle for deviations above 50Δ.

†Some surgeons prefer to limit lateral rectus muscle recessions to less than 8.0 mm These surgeons often use three-muscle surgery for deviations of 40Δ or more.

tance. In fact, it appears that bilateral lateral rectus muscle recessions equalize the distance–near disparities postoperatively as effectively as the other surgical approaches. However, one study did document better outcomes with the basic type of intermittent exotropia when a unilateral recess-resect procedure was performed.

For patients with a true high AC/A ratio, surgery is often deferred, as discussed in the section "Nonsurgical Treatment." However, satisfactory surgical results have been reported in these patients after bilateral lateral rectus muscle recession combined with bilateral medial rectus muscle posterior fixation sutures (fadenoperation).

This author's surgical plan for intermittent exotropia is presented in Table 2–2. The deviations listed in the table represent the largest deviation found on distance testing after 30 to 60 minutes of occlusion or on outdoor far distance testing. In this author's experience, children with near deviation that exceeds distance measurements are often undercorrected; therefore, 1.0 mm is added to the dosage in Table 2–2 per muscle recession. When operating on adults, the author often reduces the amount slightly to further decrease the chances of producing overcorrection and disabling diplopia. When the exodeviation measured in side gaze is 50% or less than that measured in primary position, the surgical amount is reduced by 1.0 mm per muscle to reduce the risk of overcorrection.

COMMENT

Edward G. Buckley, MD

Since the vast majority of my patients have a +3.00 D measurement that is equal to the distance measurement, either bilateral lateral rectus recessions or a medial rectus resection and lateral rectus recession could be performed. My choice for initial operation is bilateral lateral rectus recessions, only because I think that the patient is more comfortable in the immediate postoperative period. However, I agree with Dr. Wilson that in the long run, the results are equally good with a unilateral recess-resect operation.

Adjustable suture surgery can be very helpful in treating patients with intermittent exodeviation. Ideally, one would like to have a controlled slight overcorrection, which can be readily achieved with this procedure. My choice is to perform adjustable suture surgery on any patient who is old enough to tolerate it. If unilateral recess-resect procedures are performed, the adjustment becomes a bit more difficult because of the early initial overeffect of the medial rectus resection. In this case, care must be taken not to advance the recessed lateral rectus too close to the insertion during the adjustment process, as there is a definite exotropic tendency once the resected medial rectus recovers from the surgery. As an end point, I like the patient to be slightly esotropic in the primary position, with a significant esodeviation present on lateral gaze. The patient usually has a very small esodeviation in the field of the resected medial rectus as well. Care should be exercised not to adjust beyond orthophoria in the primary position, even though a significant esodeviation might persist on lateral gaze. These individuals will almost always become exotropic within 4 to 6 weeks after surgery.

COMMENT

David A. Plager, MD

I find that adjustable sutures add little to the long-term success rate for initial exotropia surgery. The problem is the highly variable initial response to similar or identical surgery among similar patients. Some patients manifest what appears to be a too large initial overcorrection in excess of 20Δ, yet spontaneously resolve to a successful outcome. Others have what appears to be an initially laudable small overcorrection, yet never straighten and require further intervention. The use of consistent surgical numbers and securing the muscle firmly to the globe provides as good or better long-term success with less discomfort than using adjustable techniques, particularly for this indication. The most important factor is managing the overcorrected patient effectively so as not to lose any fusional ability permanently.

Management of Surgical Overcorrection. A moderate (8Δ to 15Δ) temporary postoperative esodeviation is desirable after bilateral lateral rectus muscle recession. Even a large esotropia up to 25Δ in the immediate postoperative period may resolve without further surgery. Persistent overcorrection (beyond 3 or 4 weeks) may need to be treated with base-out prisms (usually Fresnel paste-on prisms) or alternate patching to prevent amblyopia or relieve diplopia. Corrective lenses or miotics are considered in cases of moderate hyperopia. Bifocals can be used if a high AC/A ratio is present. Unless deficient ductions suggest a slipped or lost muscle, a delay of 4 to 6 months is recommended before considering reoperation, because spontaneous improvement is common.

COMMENT
Edward G. Buckley, MD

Great caution should be exercised in delaying reoperation in patients with overcorrected intermittent exotropia. Preoperatively, these individuals have relatively normal binocular function with excellent stereopsis. Long periods of esotropia will result in loss of this excellent sensory condition. If a significant duction deficit is present in the field of action of the recessed lateral rectus and an esodeviation persists for more than 4 to 6 weeks, I believe that this will not resolve and intervention should be considered sooner rather than later. The muscle does not have to be *slipped* for this to occur.

COMMENT
David A. Plager, MD

Any overcorrected patient with a persistent limitation of duction is not likely to improve spontaneously and will need corrective surgery. While I agree with the admonition that one should wait 4 to 6 months for an overcorrected patient with full ductions to improve, after 2 to 3 months of persistent consecutive esotropia, I do not express much optimism to the family that this condition is likely to fully correct itself.

In children under 4 years of age, careful follow-up and aggressive use of part-time patching or prism glasses may be needed to avoid loss of high-grade stereopsis and bifixation, resulting in a secondary monofixation syndrome. Following a bilateral lateral rectus muscle recession, medial rectus muscle recessions can be performed, provided that the lateral rectus muscle ductions are normal. Unilateral lateral rectus muscle recession and medial rectus muscle resection procedures can be followed by medial rectus muscle recession and lateral rectus muscle resection on the other eye.

COMMENT
Marshall M. Parks, MD

A valid criticism of early surgery for the management of intermittent exotropia is that if overcorrection converts the strabismus to constant esotropia, amblyopia can occur. But little concern has been shown for the possibility of intermittent exotropia receiving no treatment and deteriorating to constant exotropia. Even if this latter complication occurs beyond the amblyogenic age where the monofixation no longer causes amblyopia, it permanently destroys the macular binocular vision reflex and its associated high-grade stereoacuity. This outcome cannot be considered ideal. These features make the management of intermittent exotropia more challenging than it has received credit for being.

Management of Surgical Undercorrection. Mild to moderate residual exodeviation can be left untreated and simply observed if fusional control is good. However, because manifest exotropia commonly returns with time in cases of undercorrection, some surgeons recommend treating aggressively with base-in prisms and then gradually diminishing the prism amount. Postoperative patching and orthoptic treatment using the nonsurgical techniques described previously can be effective in treating surgical undercorrection. Botulinum toxin in small doses has also been used, but data supporting its effectiveness are limited.

Indications for reoperation in undercorrected patients are the same as for the initial surgery. If lateral rectus muscle recessions were performed bilaterally, medial rectus muscle resections are often chosen when reoperation is needed. If the lateral rectus muscle recessions were 6.0 mm or less, some surgeons prefer to re-recess the lateral rectus muscles before resorting to medial rectus muscle resections. Care must be taken when re-recessing rectus muscles because the dose–response curve is steep and less predictable. Re-recession of 2.0 mm for each lateral rectus muscle may correct as much as 20Δ to 25Δ of deviation. Unilateral lateral rectus muscle recession and medial rectus muscle resection are often followed by a similar recess-resect procedure in the other eye. The surgical dose–response curve for reoperations appears to be similar to that of the initial surgery when fresh muscles are operated on. The surgical amount, therefore, can be selected as though it were a primary surgery.

COMMENT

Michael X. Repka, MD

For undercorrected intermittent exotropia, I generally perform a re-recession of the lateral rectus muscle any time the previous recession was less than 6.0 mm, combined with a medial rectus resection. I think trying to get enough effect from bilateral medial rectus resections can be very difficult, often leading to significant overcorrection at near fixation and binocular diplopia that lasts for a long time.

CONGENITAL EXOTROPIA

Congenital exotropia presents before 6 months of age as a large-angle constant exotropia (Fig. 2–4) often associated with neurologic impairment. In contrast to congenital esotropia, the incidence of congenital exotropia is low.

The potential for high-grade stereopsis and bifoveal fixation in congenital exotropia is low. Early surgery may help establish peripheral fusion. Late consecutive esotropia, recurrent exotropia, and dissociated vertical deviation are all common, even with early successful surgical alignment. A separate and distinct form of congenital exotropia can be seen in patients with various craniofacial syndromes.

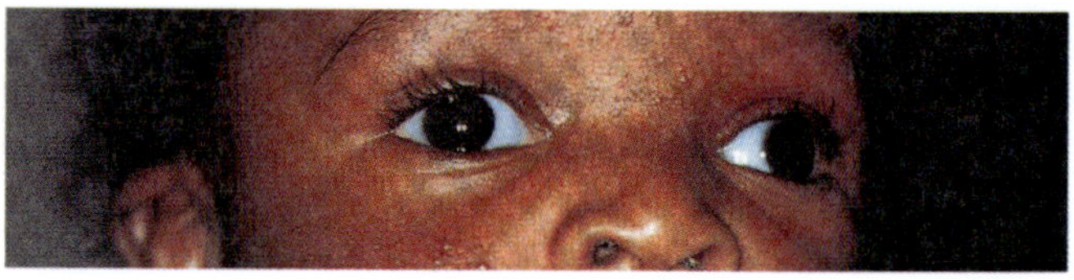

Figure 2–4. A 6-month-old infant with congenital constant exotropia.

SENSORY EXOTROPIA

Sensory exotropia, a divergent strabismus in a poorly seeing eye, can be caused by any condition that reduces visual acuity in one eye. Common causes include anisometropia, corneal or lens opacities, optic atrophy or hypoplasia, and macular lesions. It is not known why some individuals become esotropic after unilateral visual loss, while others become exotropic. Both sensory esotropia and sensory exotropia are common in young children, but exotropia predominates in older children and adults.

Because strabismus can be the presenting sign of poor visual acuity in one eye, a complete eye examination is warranted on the initial visit. Sensory strabismus, usually esotropia, is the second most common presenting sign of retinoblastoma. Oblique muscle overaction is very commonly associated with sensory strabismus, especially in the deviated eye. If the eye with sensory exotropia can be visually rehabilitated, peripheral fusion can sometimes be reestablished after surgical realignment, provided that the sensory exotropia has not been present for an extended period. Loss of fusional ability, known as *central fusional disruption*, can lead to constant and permanent diplopia when adult-onset sensory exotropia has been present for several years prior to visual rehabilitation and realignment.

CONVERGENCE INSUFFICIENCY

Patients with convergence insufficiency often present with complaints of asthenopia, blurred or diplopic near vision, and reading difficulty. Symptoms may emerge when the older child or young adult enters a level of schooling that requires prolonged reading. Burning, watery eyes and sleepiness often accompany the near visual blur, especially with fatigue. Examination reveals a remote near point of convergence and poor near fusional convergence amplitudes. An exophoria, usually present at 14 in., increases as the remote near point is reached. The eyes are well aligned for distance viewing.

The convergence insufficiency discussed here must be distinguished from the convergence insufficiency type of intermittent exotropia, in which the exotropia is present even with distant fixation but is greater with near viewing. The near point of convergence may or may not be remote, and visual blur and diplopia with reading are usually not present.

Treatment of convergence insufficiency usually involves orthoptic exercises. Base-out prism reading glasses may be used to stimulate fusional convergence. Stereograms, *pencil pushups*, and other near-point exercises are often used. If these exercises fail to improve convergence ability, base-in prism reading glasses may be needed for palliation.

Accommodative insufficiency is also present in some patients and needs to be separated from convergence insufficiency both diagnostically and therapeutically.

COMMENT

David A. Plager, MD

Surgery for convergence insufficiency can be useful for some patients, especially older adults, who are significantly troubled by their symptoms for the important near position and do not respond to nonsurgical remedies. Patients must be made aware that they may be trading near symptoms for distance ones (diplopia) and should be willing to accept that possibility. Theoretically, a unilateral medial rectus resection and a lateral rectus recession should help them adapt to any postoperative distance diplopia with a small face turn, but I think small bilateral medial rectus resections are probably a better long-term choice in the carefully selected patient who undergoes this procedure.

COMMENT

Edward G. Buckley, MD

There is a group of older individuals who develop convergence insufficiency that does not seem to be amenable to the usual orthoptic-type exercises. I have used supraplacement of the medial rectus muscles, in combination with small resections, with some success. In essence, these patients are being treated as if they had an A pattern, and supraplacing the medial rectus muscles helps create more of an effect on down gaze, as opposed to the primary position used for distance viewing. This allows small resections to become more effective for reading. The amount of supraplacement is usually a tendon width to achieve the maximal effect.

EXOTROPIC DUANE SYNDROME

Duane syndrome can present with exotropia, usually accompanied by a face turn away from the affected eye. Adduction is most often markedly deficient, and abduction is only mildly decreased. Other signs include eyelid fissure narrowing, globe retraction, and characteristic upshoots and downshoots on adduction of the affected eye.

Treatment of exotropic Duane syndrome is often more challenging than that of the more common esotropic Duane syndrome. Clinically important co-contraction and ocular upshoots and downshoots in adduction are found more commonly when primary-gaze exotropia is seen. Most authors prefer large recessions of the ipsilateral lateral rectus muscle in these patients, but this surgery further limits abduction in the operated eye and creates or increases the esotropia in lateral gaze postoperatively. Small recessions of the ipsilateral lateral rectus muscle do not result in this complication but are generally inadequate to realign the eyes in the primary position. For this reason, a very large recession (typically 10.0 mm or more) may also be needed on the contralateral lateral rectus muscle to help restore primary-position alignment.

It is the author's practice to limit recession of the ipsilateral lateral rectus muscle to the amount necessary to relieve the positive traction test for adduction. A Y-splitting procedure of the moderately recessed muscle may help eliminate upshoots and downshoots. Residual exodeviation in the primary position should then be corrected by a recession of the normal contralateral lateral rectus muscle. As stated previously, very large recessions of the normal fellow lateral rectus muscle will actually improve the field of single binocular vision by creating a duction deficit in the normal eye that may better match the residual duction deficit in the eye with Duane retraction syndrome. The addition of a posterior fixation suture on the normal fellow medial rectus muscle may also help widen the field of single binocular vision, because it will create a compensatory duction limitation in the normal eye for adduction that may match the duction limitation of the Duane retraction eye for abduction. In patients with mild exotropic Duane retraction syndrome, it may occasionally be preferable to leave the involved eye unoperated and limit surgery entirely to the normal eye.

COMMENT

Edward G. Buckley, MD

Simple recession of the involved lateral rectus will result in some improvement in the primary position but will invariably worsens the esodeviation. Thus, patients have a very small, narrow window of single binocular vision that is actually more annoying to them than their preoperative condition. Therefore, I agree with Dr. Wilson that treatment of exotropic Duane syndrome patients involves mainly surgery on the normal eye. The only time I operate on the involved eye is for significant retraction on attempted adduction or an upshoot or downshoot. In my experience, it is extremely difficult to cripple the contralateral lateral rectus muscle enough to balance the forces, so the amount of recession is in excess of 12.0 to 15.0 mm. It is almost impossible to overcorrect this condition.

Suggested Readings

Biedner B, Marcus M, David R, et al: Congenital constant exotropia: surgical results in six patients. *Binocul Vis Eye Muscle Surg Q* 1993; 8:137–140.

Brodsky MC, Fray KJ: Surgical management of intermittent exotropia with high AC/A ratio. *J Am Assoc Pediatr Ophthalmol Strabismus* 1998; 2:330–332.

Burian HM, Spivey BE: The surgical management of exodeviations. *Am J Ophthalmol* 1965; 59:603–620.

Caltrider N, Jampolsky A: Overcorrecting minus lens therapy for treatment of intermittent exotropia. *Ophthalmology* 1983; 90:1160–1165.

Coffey B, Wick B, Cotter S, et al: Treatment options in intermittent exotropia: a critical appraisal. *Optom Vis Sci* 1992; 69:386–404.

Cooper J, Medow N: Major review: intermittent exotropia; basic and divergence excess type. *Binocul Vis Eye Muscle Surg Q* 1993; 8:185–216.

Costenbader FD: The physiology and management of divergent strabismus. In: Allen JH, ed: *Symposium on Strabismus: Transactions of the New Orleans Academy of Ophthalmology*. St Louis: CV Mosby Co; 1950:349–366.

Freeman RS, Isenberg SJ: The use of part-time occlusion for early onset unilateral exotropia. *J Pediatr Ophthalmol Strabismus* 1989; 26:94–96.

Havertape SA, Cruz OA, Chu FC: Sensory strabismus—eso or exo? *J Pediatr Ophthalmol Strabismus* 2001; 38:327–330.

Hunter DG, Ellis FJ: Prevalence of systemic and ocular disease in infantile exotropia: comparison with infantile esotropia. *Ophthalmology* 1999; 106:1951–1956.

Iacobucci IL, Archer SM, Giles CL: Children with exotropia responsive to spectacle correction of hyperopia. *Am J Ophthalmol* 1993; 116:79–83.

Kushner BJ: Exotropic deviations: a functional classification and approach to treatment. *Am Orthopt J* 1998; 38:81–93.

Kushner BJ: Selective surgery for intermittent exotropia based on distance/near differences. *Arch Ophthalmol* 1998; 116:324–328.

Kushner BJ: Diagnosis and treatment of exotropia with a high accommodation convergence–accommodation ratio. *Arch Ophthalmol* 1999; 117:221–224.

Kushner BJ: Does overcorrecting minus lens therapy for intermittent exotropia cause myopia? *Arch Ophthalmol* 1999; 117:638–642.

Moore S: The prognostic value of lateral gaze measurements in intermittent exotropia. *Am Orthopt J* 1969; 19:69–71.

Nelson LB, Calhoun JH, Harley RD, eds: *Pediatric Ophthalmology*, 3rd ed. Philadelphia: WB Saunders Co; 1991.

Repka MX, Arnoldi KA: Lateral incomitance in exotropia: fact or artifact? *J Pediatr Ophthalmol Strabismus* 1991; 28:125–128; discussion 129–130.

Rosenbaum AL: Evaluation and management of intermittent exotropia. *Am Orthopt J* 1996; 46:94–98.

Saunders RA, Wilson ME, Bluestein EC, et al: Surgery on the normal eye in Duane retraction syndrome. *J Pediatr Ophthalmol Strabismus* 1994; 31:162–169; discussion 170–171.

Wiggins RE, von Noorden GK: Monocular eye closure in sunlight. *J Pediatr Ophthalmol Strabismus* 1990; 27:16–20; discussion 21–22.

Wilson ME, Parks MM: Primary inferior oblique overaction in congenital esotropia, accommodative esotropia, and intermittent exotropia. *Ophthalmology* 1989; 96:950–955; discussion 956–957.

3

Oblique Muscle Dysfunction

DAVID A. PLAGER

The inferior and superior oblique muscles can cause strabismus by either underacting or overacting. It may be more precise to call these eye movement abnormalities *overelevation in adduction*, *underdepression in abduction*, and so on, stressing the result, not the cause, but the terms *underaction* and *overaction* to describe oblique muscle dysfunction are so ingrained in our lexicon that these clinically descriptive terms are used in the chapter. These underactions and overactions are usually graded relative to the duction of the opposite eye and are conventionally termed either *primary* or *secondary*—to paresis or restriction of ipsilateral antagonist muscles or dysfunction in the opposite eye.

Clinically apparent primary underactions, when not caused by a restrictive process in the eye, are usually due to either a nerve paresis/paralysis or an anatomic anomaly (Fig. 3–1). Secondary underactions are not a clinically relevant problem.

Although the term *overaction* is used commonly in strabismus, primary overaction of an oblique muscle on the basis of hyperfunction of the muscle is hard to rationalize. The many theories offered to explain primary oblique muscle overaction are a testament to our lack of firm understanding of this entity. There is little reason to think that these muscles are overinnervated, although recent work has suggested that some primary oblique muscle overaction is caused by vestibular dysfunction and is related to the primitive ocular reflexes of lateral-eyed animals.

Many oblique muscle overactions are obviously secondary overactions. These may be secondary to underaction or paresis of the ipsilateral antagonist muscle—for example, the inferior oblique overaction that is common with superior oblique palsy—or they may be secondary to a deficiency or restriction of movement in the opposite eye—for example, the inferior oblique overaction seen in an eye whose fellow eye has an up-gaze restriction.

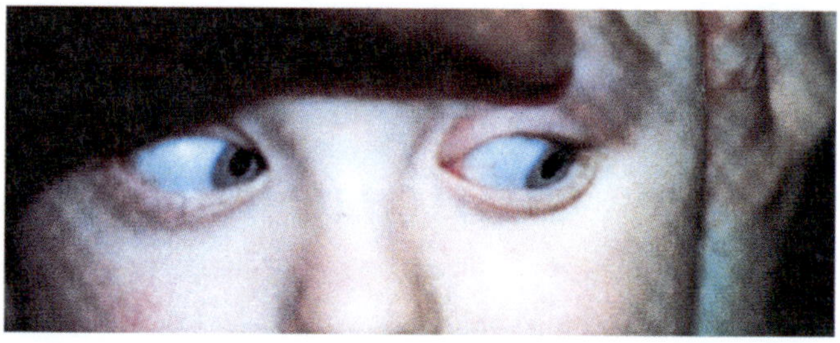

A

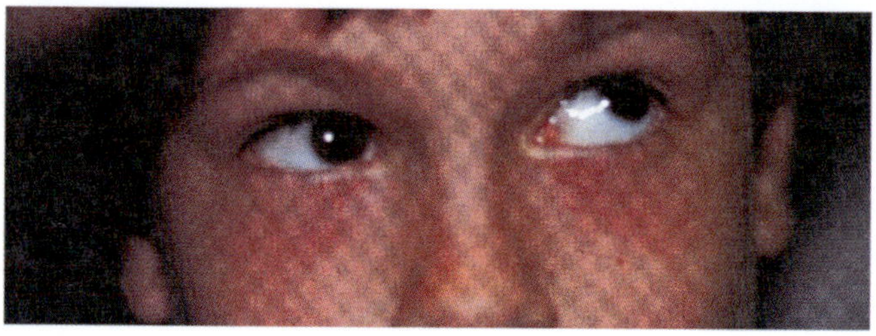

B

Figure 3–1. Underactions of oblique muscles. (*A*) Superior oblique underaction in superior oblique palsy. (*B*) Inferior oblique underaction in inferior oblique palsy.

CAUSES OF OBLIQUE MUSCLE OVERACTION

Apparent oblique muscle overaction, that is, overelevation or overdepression of the adducted eye, can be caused by muscle anomaly, orbit abnormality, adduction deficiency, or innervation anomaly or can be secondary to restriction in the fellow eye. Clinical examples of these causes are described in the sections that follow.

Muscle Anomaly. Inferior oblique overaction can be caused by the *underchecking* phenomenon from a lax or, rarely, absent superior oblique tendon (Fig. 3–2). This is frequently found unilaterally in cases of congenital superior oblique palsy, but can also be found bilaterally in cases of bilateral overaction with a V pattern.

Superior oblique overaction from an anomalous inferior oblique muscle is not a clinically known condition except in cases of iatrogenic superior oblique overaction following surgical weakening of the inferior oblique muscle.

Orbit Abnormality. Also known as *pulley heterotopia*, apparent oblique overaction can be due to heterotopic rectus muscle pulleys. This causes relative upshoots or downshoots in adduction. This entity can be suspected on clinical grounds, including facial/orbital appearance, but requires orbital imaging to confirm. Craniofacial dysostoses, such as Crouzon syndrome, provide extreme examples of this phenomenon (Fig. 3–3).

Underaction of the ipsilateral antagonist oblique muscle is also present in these cases, and surgical weakening of the overacting oblique muscle is usually ineffective. Vertical shifts of the horizontal rectus muscles help correct the underlying cause of the abnormality.

A
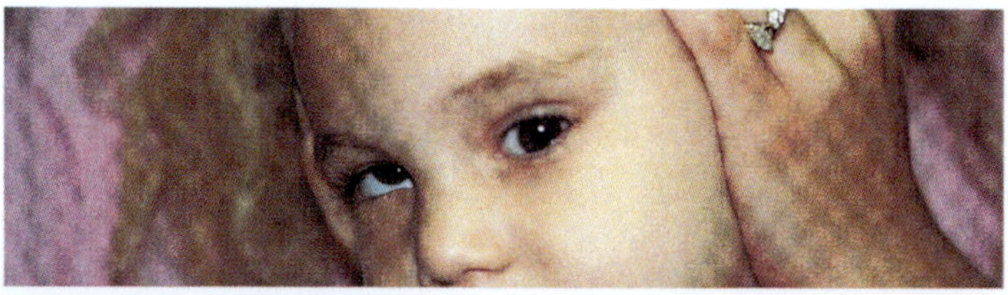

B
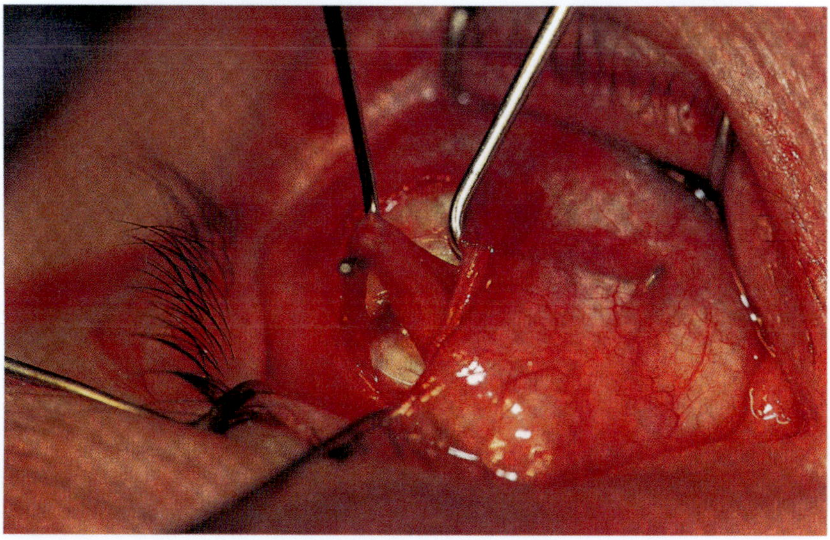

Figure 3–2. Inferior oblique overaction can occur secondary to *underchecking* of the antagonist superior oblique when the superior oblique tendon is excessively lax, as in congenital superior oblique palsy. (*A*) Right inferior oblique overaction secondary to congenital superior oblique palsy with (*B*) a lax superior oblique tendon.

Adduction Deficiency. Apparent overaction of both oblique muscles in the same eye, with a resultant X pattern, may be present in cases of adduction deficiency (Fig. 3–4). This may be seen primarily in cases of large-angle exotropia or secondarily after medial rectus recession, especially if the recession is excessive or complicated by the slipped-muscle phenomenon. In these cases, the oblique dysfunction is cured by fixing the adduction limitation and does not require surgery on the oblique muscles.

COMMENT

Edward G. Buckley, MD

True overaction can be distinguished from pseudo-overaction in large-angle exotropia by making an assessment on lateral gaze. A significant hyperdeviation will be present in true overaction, whereas in pseudo-overaction, some vertical movement is usually necessary to cause the oblique to pull excessively.

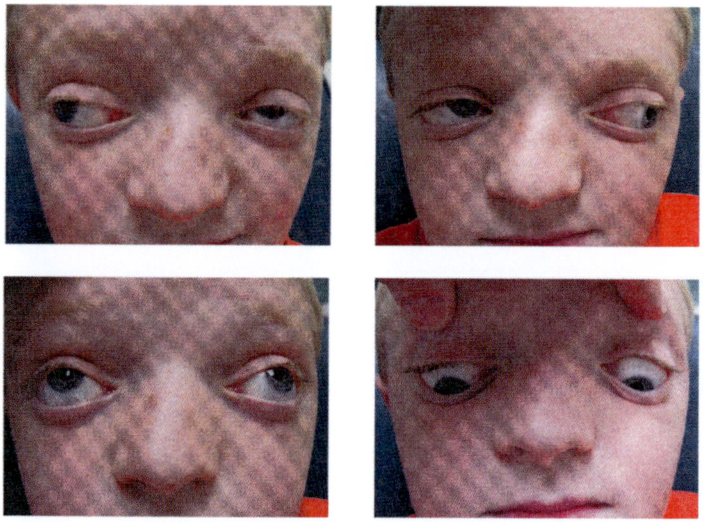

A

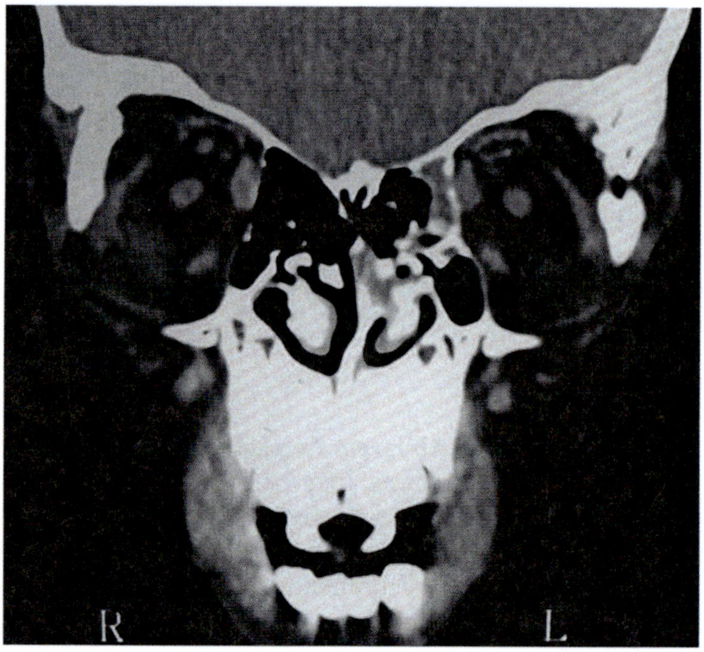

B

Figure 3–3. Orbit abnormality. (*A*) Cranial facial syndrome (Crouzon) and large V-pattern exotropia associated with overelevation in adduction. (*B*) Magnetic resonance imaging scan of a similar patient showing pulley heterotopy. Note the relative supraplacement of the medial rectus muscles relative to the lateral rectus muscles and excyclorotation of the oribts.

Innervation Anomaly. A secondary oblique overaction will follow nerve insult, that is, palsy of the antagonist oblique muscle. For instance, inferior oblique overaction is common in cases of superior oblique palsy, and superior oblique overaction can be seen secondary to inferior oblique palsy.

An unrelated innervation anomaly, Duane syndrome, can be associated with upshoots and downshoots in adduction as the globe slides above or below the tight lateral rectus muscle (Fig. 3–5).

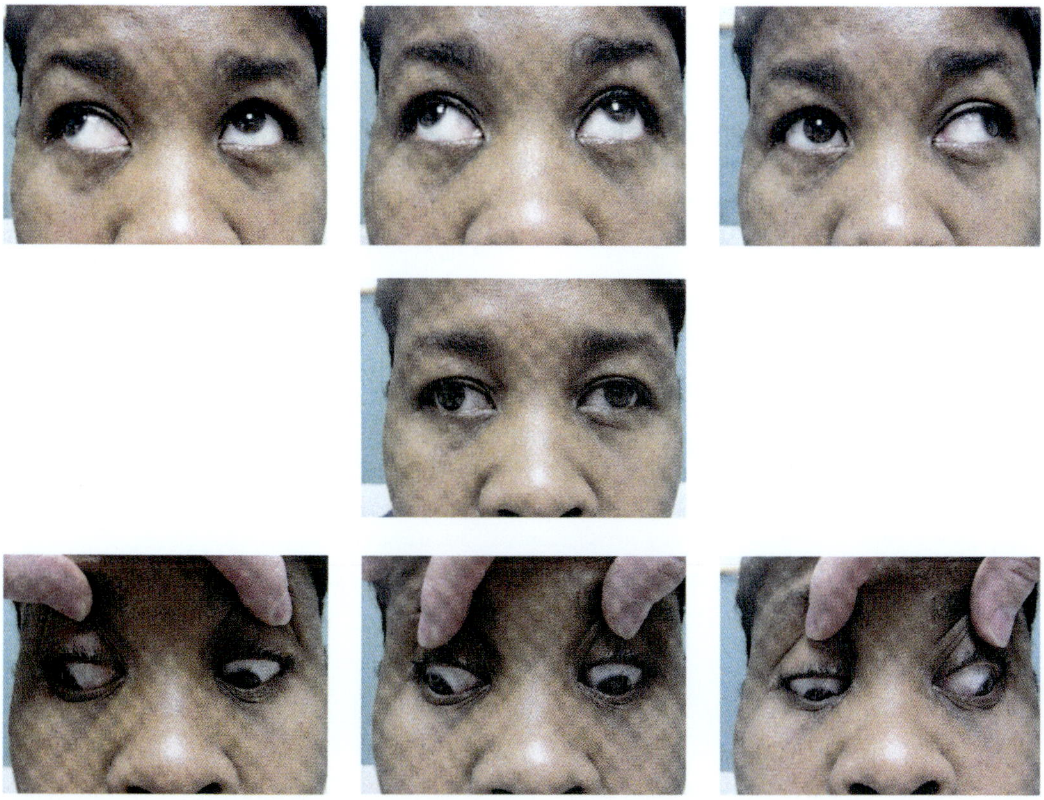

Figure 3–4. Relative overelevation in adduction secondary to large-angle exotropia. Note what appears to be both bilateral inferior oblique and superior oblique overaction with a resultant X pattern. Correcting the horizontal deviation will diminish the oblique dysfunction and eliminate the X pattern.

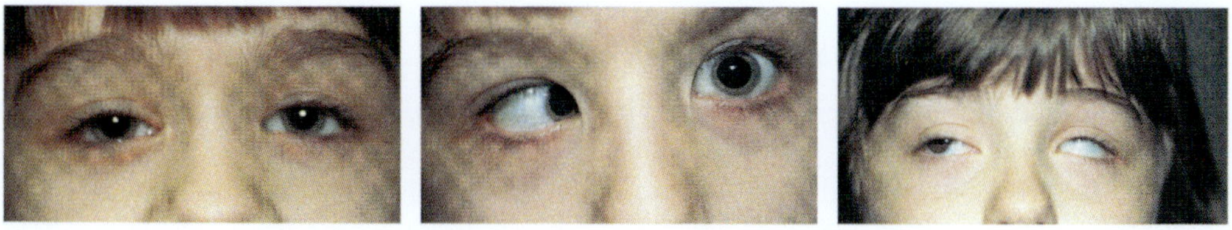

A B C

Figure 3–5. Overelevation in adduction caused by the upshoot phenomenon associated with Duane syndrome. (*A*) Primary position. (*B*) Absent abduction of left eye on left gaze. (*C*) Marked upshoot of the left eye on right gaze (cornea elevated above the upper lid margin).

Contralateral Restriction. Overelevation in adduction can be apparent when there is an elevation deficiency in the opposite eye (Fig. 3–6). Common conditions causing this entity include inferior rectus entrapment following orbital floor blowout fracture, inferior rectus restriction from thyroid ophthalmopathy, double elevator palsy (monocular elevation deficiency), and iatrogenic results of ophthalmic or sinus surgery. In this case, surgical attention is usually best focused on relieving the condition in the fellow eye.

INFERIOR OBLIQUE OVERACTION

Inferior oblique overaction can be secondary to any of the five causes discussed earlier: muscle anomaly, orbit abnormality, adduction deficiency, innervation anomaly, or contralateral restriction. Inferior oblique overaction not secondary to

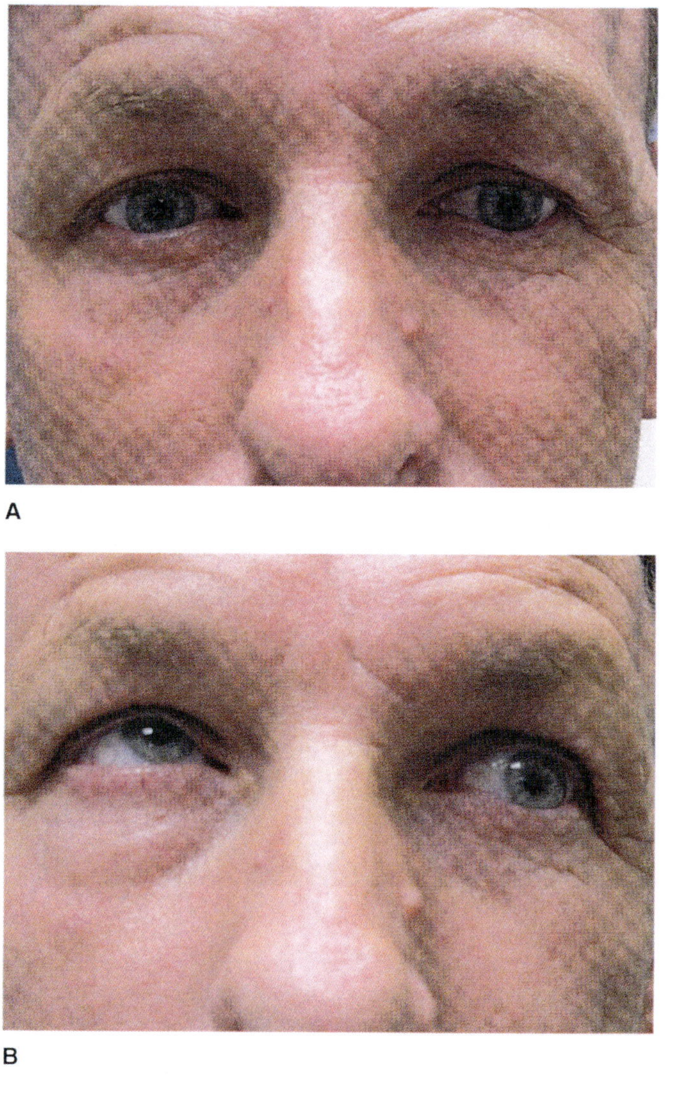

A

B

Figure 3–6. Overelevation in adduction caused by restriction of elevation in the opposite eye. Common causes include inferior orbital floor (blowout) fracture, asymmetric thyroid disease, inferior oblique adherence or inclusion syndromes, and unilateral (contralateral) inferior oblique anterior transposition. (*A*) Left hypotropia in primary position. (*B*) Overaction of the right inferior oblique secondary to restricted elevation of the left eye.

one of those causes is termed *primary overaction*, which is found most commonly as part of the congenital esotropia complex (see Chapter 1, "Esotropic Deviations"). Many, but not all, cases of inferior oblique overaction in congenital esotropia are found in patients with abnormal laxity of the superior oblique tendons, and this could be considered overaction secondary to an underchecking of these lax superior obliques.

COMMENT

Gunter K. von Noorden, MD

Some medical terms outlive their usefulness and need to be modified or replaced when they are no longer correct. This pertains to the diagnosis-laden *overaction or underaction of the inferior or superior oblique muscles.* As pointed out in this chapter, many conditions may be responsible for overelevation or overdepression of an adducted eye. However, only secondary deviations following paralysis of the ipsilateral antagonist or of the contralateral yoke muscle account for true overaction, that is, increased innervation of a muscle. True primary overaction of an oblique muscle apart from these conditions has not been well understood, and whether it exists at all has become increasingly doubtful.

Diagnosis. Diagnosis of inferior oblique overaction is made by recognition of an overelevation of the involved eye in adduction compared to the fellow eye in abduction. The degree of overaction is typically graded on a 1+ to 4+ scale, which corresponds to approximately 5 to 20 prism diopters (Δ) of hypertropia of the involved eye in the field of action of the inferior oblique.

Surgical Treatment. Treatment considerations for secondary overaction of the inferior oblique are covered in the sections discussing the causes of the secondary overaction. Primary overaction of the inferior oblique should be treated when it causes a significant V pattern or when it is otherwise objectionable. In general, 1+ overaction is rarely treated, 2+ is sometimes treated, 3+ is frequently treated, and 4+ is almost always treated. There are no nonsurgical treatment alternatives.

Many surgical procedures for weakening the inferior oblique have been described, including graded recession, anteriorization, myectomy, disinsertion, denervation, extirpation, and Z myotomy. Of these, graded recession, myectomy, and anteriorization are the most common procedures performed today.

Graded recession. Some surgeons prefer to weaken the inferior oblique by graded recession after Parks, usually a so-called 10.0 mm recession for mild (2+) overaction and a 14.0 mm recession for moderate (3+) overaction. Unlike rectus muscle recessions, inferior oblique recessions are not quantified intraoperatively. Instead, these recession points are identified by the consistent anatomic landmarks in the inferior temporal quadrant of the globe. The 10.0 mm recession point for reattachment of the inferior oblique is a mark placed 3.0 mm posterior and

2.0 mm temporal to the lateral border of the inferior rectus. The 14.0 mm recession point straddles the exit from the globe of the inferior temporal vortex vein along the lateral border of the inferior rectus (Fig. 3–7).

One advantage of a recession is that the surgeon has reliable knowledge of where the inferior oblique can be found, should the need arise for reoperation on that muscle. In addition, a small recession may be less prone to overcorrection than other weakening procedures for mild degrees of inferior oblique overaction. These attributes make reoperation on an overly weakened inferior oblique theoretically easier following recession than myectomy, but practically, this is not a significant advantage.

Myectomy. Another large group of surgeons favors myectomy for inferior oblique weakening of all degrees of overaction. Myectomy is thought to be a self-grading procedure that produces the amount of effect needed in most cases. Although many techniques are available, the author prefers to perform a complete myectomy by excising all of the sub-Tenon's portion of the muscle between the insertion and the Tenon's penetration site (Fig. 3–8). This eliminates any chance of reanastomosis of the transected muscle ends, since the distal end is excised. The Tenon's penetration site can be closed with an 8-0 absorbable suture, but there is insufficient evidence that this additional step is more effective.

Denervation and extirpation. The denervation and extirpation procedure is favored by some as the most powerful weakening procedure for markedly (4+) overactive muscles. This extirpation is really a supermaximal myectomy, since the proximal portion of the inferior oblique remains. With denervation alone, there is a nearly 100% rate of recurrence of the inferior oblique overaction. In this combined procedure, the transection of the nerve to the inferior oblique allows access to a larger section of the inferior oblique muscle for myectomy and excision (Fig. 3–9). There is some controversy as to whether this additional step produces a greater effect than conventional myectomy.

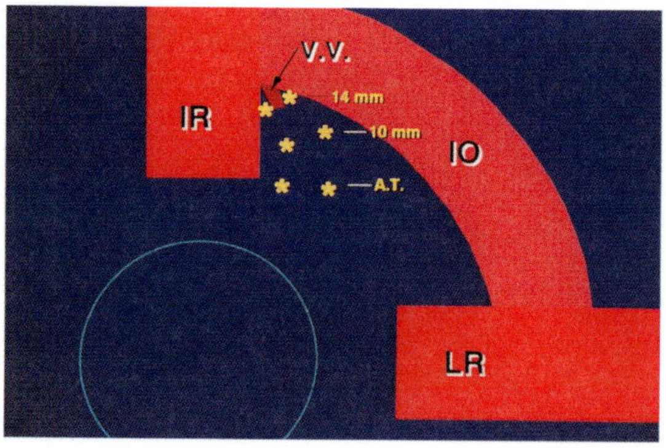

Figure 3–7. Three common reattachment points for graded inferior oblique (IO) recession: the 10.0 mm recession point is 3.0 mm posterior and 2.0 mm lateral to the lateral border of the inferior rectus (IR) insertion; the 14.0 mm recession site straddles the vortex vein (VV) in the inferior temporal quadrant; the anterior transposition (AT) site is adjacent and just anterior to the lateral border of the inferior rectus insertion. LR = lateral rectus.

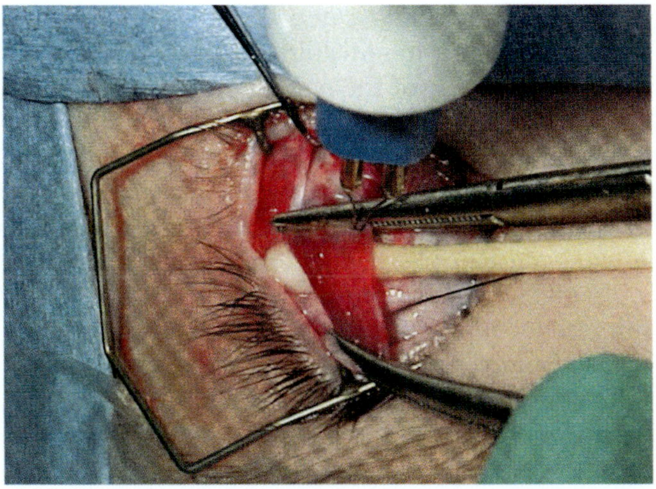

Figure 3–8. Myectomy. Hot cautery can be used judiciously to cut and cauterize sub-Tenon's portion of muscle. Care must be taken not to touch any other structures with the cautery. A cotton swab is placed under the muscle to protect the globe.

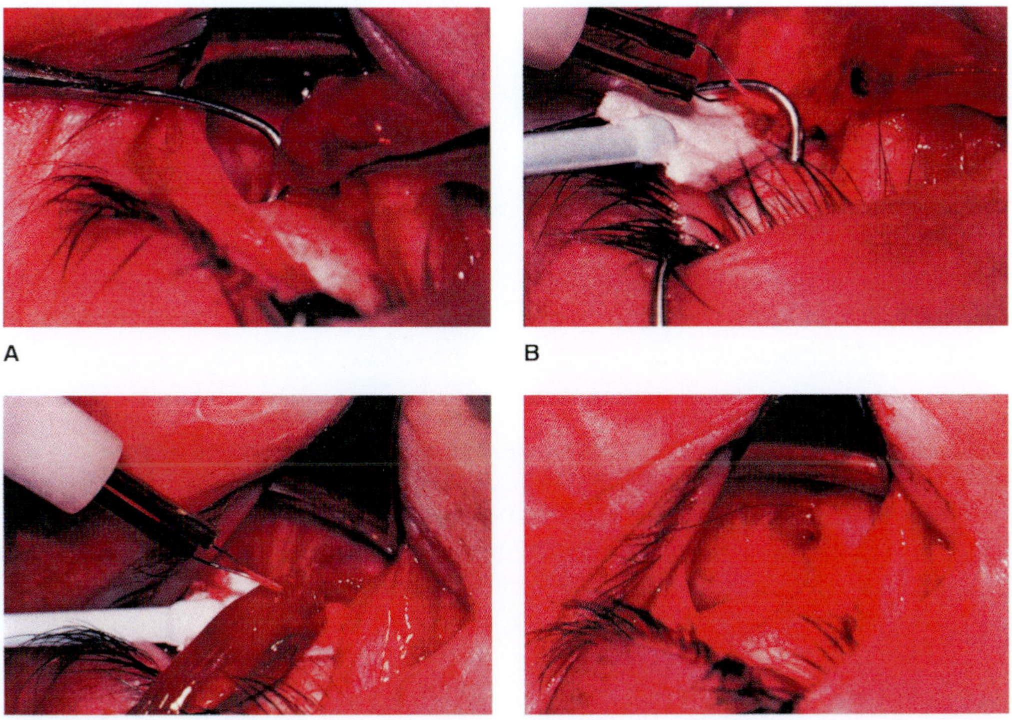

A B C D

Figure 3–9. If desired, the nerve to the inferior oblique can be identified and transected prior to clamping and transecting the muscle. This allows for a larger portion of the inferior muscle to be resected, the so-called denervation/extirpation procedure of Parks. (*A*) The nerve to the inferior oblique is hooked with a Stevens hook. (*B*) The nerve is transected with a hot cautery, which allows the muscle to spring forward. (*C*) A large section of the inferior oblique can be tied off and resected. (*D*) The remaining stump of the inferior oblique is pushed back through Tenon's capsule.

Anterior transposition. Also called *anteriorization*, anterior transposition of the insertion of the inferior oblique is a significant modification of the recession procedure. Anteriorization refers to the placement of the new insertion just anterior and adjacent to the temporal border of the inferior rectus insertion. This point is anterior to the equator of the eye and should, theoretically, change the inferior oblique from an elevator of the eye to a depressor. In reality, because of the other intermuscular connections and because the inferior oblique is not innervated on attempted down gaze, the anteriorized inferior oblique does not depress the eye, but this is a very powerful inferior oblique weakening procedure.

Anteriorization of the inferior oblique produces a relative restriction to up gaze in the operated eye. This is not readily apparent when the procedure is performed bilaterally, but it is apparent when performed unilaterally. Therefore, this procedure should not be performed unilaterally except in the unusual situation where the surgeon intends to create an asymmetric restriction.

Because of the variable incomitance and relative restriction, this procedure is not recommended for treatment of superior oblique palsy or other conditions typically associated with the potential for high degrees of binocular function. In contrast, induced up-gaze restriction can be beneficial in patients with dissociated vertical deviation associated with inferior oblique overaction. The combination of inferior oblique overaction with dissociated vertical deviation is the prime indication for anterior transposition of the inferior oblique. It is also reasonable to use this procedure prophylactically in children with bilateral inferior oblique overaction who are at risk for developing dissociated vertical deviation later as part of the congenital (infantile) esotropia complex.

COMMENT

Edward G. Buckley, MD

After aggressive inferior oblique anteriorization, a restriction of elevation in abduction of that eye occurs (antielevation syndrome). This will appear as contralateral inferior oblique overaction. Because the restriction of elevation in abduction is greater than the limitation of elevation in adduction, persistently overacting inferior obliques can occur after bilateral inferior oblique anteriorization, due to this antielevation syndrome rather than to failure to weaken adequately the inferior oblique muscle. When this occurs unilaterally, the treatment is to reverse the anteriorization rather than weakening the contralateral inferior oblique. When it occurs bilaterally, both inferior obliques need to be unanteriorized.

COMMENT

M. Edward Wilson, MD

In my view, the 14.0 mm inferior oblique muscle recession is less effective than the 10.0 mm recession. The classic 3.0 mm back and 2.0 mm over position of the 10.0 mm recession gives it some anteriorization effect. The 14.0 mm recession position is more difficult to reach and may not offer any advantages over the 10.0 mm recession. Since myectomy works for 1+ to 4+ overaction (you get what you need), grading of recessions based on the severity of the inferior oblique muscle overaction may be unnecessary. I suggest that surgeons apply the 10.0 mm recession or the myectomy (surgeon's preference—I like the recession better since it can be altered more easily later if needed) for all degrees of severity of inferior oblique overaction. The anterior transposition should be applied when dissociated vertical deviation is also being treated.

INFERIOR OBLIQUE UNDERACTION

Palsy. Inferior oblique underaction, clinically manifest as a deficiency of elevation in adduction, can be due to inferior oblique palsy/paresis or to a restrictive process such as Brown syndrome (discussed below).

Theoretically, isolated palsy of the inferior oblique should be quite rare, since it requires damage to a single branch of the inferior division of the oculomotor nerve without affecting the other branches that supply the medial rectus and the pupil. However, the condition seems to occur more commonly than might be expected on a purely neuroanatomic basis, developing in both children and adults.

Patients present with a vertical deviation, usually small, and frequently a head tilt. Symptoms may include diplopia or asthenopia.

Diagnosis. The diagnosis is made by applying Parks' three-step test to a hypertropia that is measured to be greatest in horizontal gaze toward the opposite eye and head tilt toward the opposite eye. For example, a right hypertropia that increases on right gaze and right head tilt would incriminate the left inferior oblique as paretic.

Double Maddox rod testing may show incyclotorsion, although commonly no torsion is uncovered. A finding of subjective excyclotorsion should cause the diagnosis to be questioned and the case reevaluated (Fig. 3–10).

In the absence of other localizing clinical signs or symptoms, neurologic evaluation or neuroimaging is unlikely to be helpful and is not indicated for isolated inferior oblique palsy.

COMMENT

Michael X. Repka, MD

In a patient in whom I am considering the diagnosis of isolated inferior oblique paresis, I carefully examine the pupil for the response to light and near, as well as looking for signs of aberrant regeneration. These are usually easiest to see by watching as the eyes move from adduction to abduction and from primary position to down gaze.

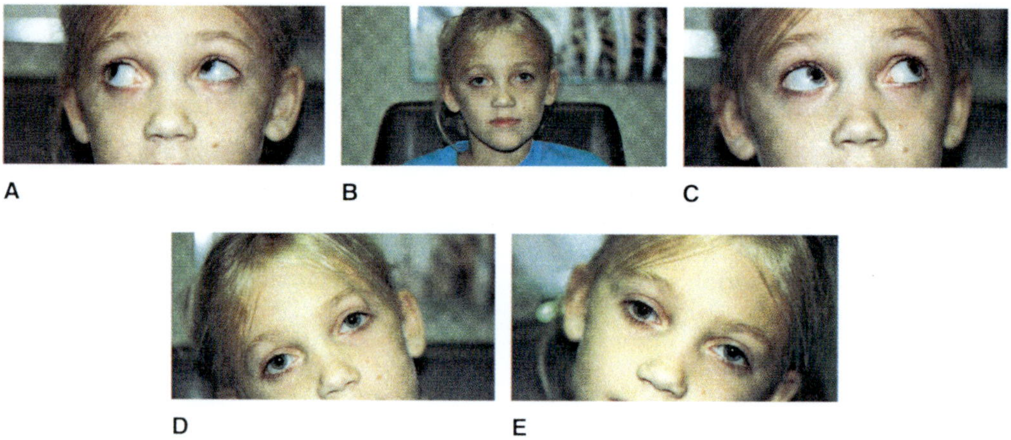

Figure 3–10A–E. Right inferior oblique palsy. Three-step test measurements will show hypertropia that increases on gaze and head tilt opposite to the side of the affected muscle. Incyclotorsion should be present on double Maddox rod testing.

Differential diagnosis. The diagnosis most often confused with paresis of the inferior oblique is a mild Brown syndrome, a restrictive process of the superior oblique complex (discussed below). Moderate and severe Brown syndrome are more clinically apparent. In the clinic, one may be able to differentiate the paretic inferior oblique from the restricted superior oblique by measuring differential intraocular pressure between primary gaze and up gaze or by performing forced duction testing if the patient is willing, though usually these maneuvers are not necessary. Ultimately, these two clinical processes are usually distinguished in the operating room with traction testing of the superior oblique. Brown syndrome is confirmed by a markedly tight superior oblique tendon.

COMMENT

Edward G. Buckley, MD

Most of the time, inferior oblique paresis can be distinguished from Brown syndrome in the clinic. While both cause an elevation defect in adduction of the involved eye, inferior oblique paresis is associated with an A pattern, incyclotorsion, an overacting superior oblique, and a positive head-tilt test. Brown syndrome usually has a V pattern, no torsion, a negative head-tilt test, and minimal overaction of the superior oblique. Of these factors, the A and V patterns seem to be the most consistent and most easily observable conditions that enable differentiation between these two entities.

Surgical treatment. Although small comitant deviations may be amenable to prism treatment with spectacles, surgery is usually indicated in patients for whom prisms are not a successful or viable option. For small to moderate deviations of up to 15Δ in the primary position, recession of the yoke superior rectus muscle of the opposite eye is the most reliable and safe procedure.

A weakening procedure of the ipsilateral superior oblique can be considered, but it should be reserved for patients with particularly large deviations and significant degrees of incyclotorsion. Superior oblique weakening in a fusing patient without incyclotorsion should be avoided.

COMMENT

Marshall M. Parks, MD

Inferior oblique hypofunction that gradually appears in an older child or adult and is diagnostically confirmed by the three-step test as inferior oblique palsy troubles me. Its nerve fibers within the third (oculomotor) nerve are difficult to comprehend as the only ones discretely involved. In addition, my experience with its reinnervation that invariably so rapidly follows surgical denervation, with return of full function, adds to my doubt about this diagnosis.

The author mentions that the diagnosis most often confused with inferior oblique paresis is ipsilateral Brown syndrome, but the Bielschowsky head-tilt test measurements are always negative in Brown syndrome, whereas they are positive in inferior oblique palsy. Although I remain uneasy about making this diagnosis, I admit that the diagnostic facts presented by the three-step test—a test designed to make the diagnosis of a palsied, isolated cyclovertical muscle—cannot be dismissed out of hand. Yet I have been sufficiently troubled by this diagnosis to have suggested that possibly the correct diagnosis is primary overaction of the ipsilateral superior oblique. However, this suggestion remains unproven. When incyclodeviation is present in the primary position, combined with the vertical deviation, I tenotomize the superior oblique tendon and insert a 6.0 mm silicone spacer. If cyclodeviation is lacking, weakening the yoke superior rectus muscle is the safest procedure.

Brown Syndrome. The term *Brown syndrome* is used to describe an eye with deficient elevation in adduction due to restriction of the superior oblique tendon or the trochlea–tendon complex. The original theory ascribing the elevation deficiency to an anomalous tendon sheath has long been abandoned, but the precise mechanism of the restriction remains an enigma and is probably multifactorial. Brown syndrome can be congenital or acquired, unilateral (90%) or bilateral (10%).

One hypothesis, though unproven, is that at least some cases of congenital Brown syndrome lie on a continuum with congenital superior oblique palsy. In the former, the tendon is too short; in the latter, too long. Restrictions due to these tight tendons can be relieved by surgically lengthening the tendon. Yet some cases of congenital Brown syndrome have been known to resolve spontaneously, implying a temporary restriction in the trochlea–tendon relationship, not a permanently short tendon.

Histopathologic evidence implies that the tendon does not slide through the trochlea like a rope through a pulley; instead, the tendon has a telescoping mechanism as the adjacent tendon fibers slide past each other, with the trochlea acting to redirect the direction of pull. If the pathology were always confined to the trochlea–sheath complex, corrective surgery would not normalize the superior oblique function simply by lengthening the tendon. The author has seen one case of acute-onset superior oblique palsy in a child that evolved over several months to a typical-appearing Brown syndrome in the same eye. The pathophysiology of such a transformation is unexplained.

COMMENT

M. Edward Wilson, MD

> There is no histopathologic evidence for the assertion that the superior oblique tendon is short in congenital Brown syndrome. Congenital, acquired, constant, and intermittent Brown syndrome are part of the same spectrum. Although other conditions can masquerade as Brown syndrome, classic Brown syndrome is caused by a stenosis in the trochlear complex. The superior oblique tendon is normal. If it were short, it would likely be overacting and would not result in superior oblique muscle palsy after it was lengthened.

Children with congenital Brown syndrome may present with inability to elevate an eye, torticollis (which characteristically involves a chin-up posture with face turn to the opposite side), or just the observation that the two eyes "don't move together."

Cases of typical congenital Brown syndrome seldom require neuroimaging or other systemic evaluation. Scans performed in the search for masses, cysts, or other anatomic abnormalities rarely facilitate the diagnosis or treatment.

Acquired Brown syndrome may look similar to the congenital variety, but the possible causes are more varied. Brown syndrome can be acquired following eye surgery either directly on the superior oblique, such as an excessive tuck, or indirectly by inserting foreign bodies, such as a glaucoma valve or scleral buckling hardware, in the region of the superior oblique. Acquired Brown syndrome can also occur secondary to inflammatory, infectious, or traumatic processes in the trochlear region.

Older children and adults with acquired Brown syndrome may note intermittent diplopia and perhaps pain or tenderness with eye movement or digital pressure over the trochlear region.

Workup of an acquired Brown syndrome should include neuroimaging of the orbits, with attention to the trochlea, and any systemic evaluation suggested by associated constitutional symptoms, such as arthritis or another connective tissue disease. Many, perhaps most, cases of acquired Brown syndrome are not explained by the results of neuroimaging or systemic evaluation.

COMMENT
Edward G. Buckley, MD

Neuroimaging in acquired Brown syndrome, while always recommended, rarely provides useful information. I do not recall seeing a positive computed tomography (CT) scan in these individuals. The greatest yield is achieved by careful palpation of the trochlear area. In acute inflammatory cases, this area is almost always somewhat swollen and tender. While the literature reports a significant association between acquired Brown syndrome and rheumatoid arthritis, in actuality most of the workups in this disorder are negative.

Diagnosis. The diagnosis is made by recognition of a significant deficiency of elevation in adduction. The patient may have a hypotropia in the involved eye and a head tilt (with a chin-up posture) that is usually away from the involved side (Fig. 3–11). The elevation deficiency is most marked in adduction, is less apparent in up gaze, and may be nearly normal in abduction.

Differential diagnosis. The restrictive up-gaze deficiency of Brown syndrome must be differentiated from a paretic deficiency of the inferior oblique. Brown syndrome usually has little or no superior oblique overaction and is frequently associated with a V pattern. Superior oblique traction testing definitively separates these two entities by disclosing the markedly restricted up gaze with Brown syndrome.

Other up-gaze deficiencies should be apparent by examination or history. Double elevator palsy (monocular elevation deficiency) shows similarly deficient up gaze in abduction and adduction and is invariably associated with ptosis.

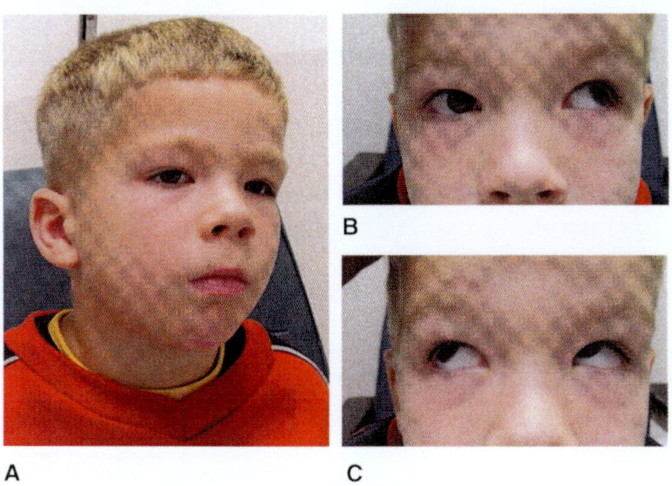

Figure 3–11. Brown syndrome. (*A*) Head posture is frequently chin-up, with tilt away from the side of the lesion. (*B*) Marked underelevation in adduction of the right eye. (*C*) Normal elevation in adduction of the left eye.

Congenital fibrosis of the inferior rectus or multiple rectus muscles can also cause an up-gaze deficiency across all up-gaze positions and usually has associated ptosis. Attempted up gaze usually results in esotropia, whereas up gaze in Brown syndrome usually results in a splaying out of the eye, giving an exotropia with the appearance of a V pattern.

Other inferior restrictive problems, such as blowout fracture, thyroid-related ophthalmopathy, and surgical or other trauma, should be readily apparent by the history and associated findings.

Surgical treatment. Surgery for Brown syndrome is usually done for unacceptable head posture or diplopia. In general, treatment is similar to that of other restrictive strabismus entities: to treat the condition successfully, the restriction needs to be relieved. In this case, surgery is usually directed at elongating the shortened superior oblique tendon. Partial weakening procedures of the superior oblique tendon are ineffective for all but the most minor elevation restrictions. Patients with mild Brown syndrome usually do not require surgery. As children grow taller, the implications of their up-gaze deficiency lessen.

Once the diagnosis is confirmed by superior oblique traction testing, the restriction must be relieved by a complete severing (tenotomy) of the superior oblique tendon. The author prefers to do this nasal to the superior rectus after approaching the tendon through a fornix incision temporal to the superior rectus, as described by Parks. It is imperative that traction testing be repeated after severing of the tendon to confirm completeness of the tenotomy and freeing of the elevation restriction.

Although a free tenotomy of the superior oblique tendon can relieve the elevation restriction, this procedure may be complicated by development of a secondary superior oblique paresis in a significant percentage of patients. To decrease the incidence of superior oblique paresis following tenotomy in Brown syndrome, several guarded tenotomy procedures, including suspending the cut edges of the tendon with a loop of suture, have been described.

Wright described placement of a section of silicone band used for scleral buckling procedures between the cut ends of the tendon. This rigid structure allows for a graded lengthening of the superior oblique tendon while simultaneously preventing the ends from separating too far, therefore decreasing the incidence of secondary superior oblique underaction.

The appropriate length of silicone spacer is determined intraoperatively based on the relative tightness of the superior oblique tendon. At least 5.0 mm is necessary to affect a clinically relevant Brown syndrome. Spacers longer than 7.0 mm are more likely to extrude and should normally be avoided.

COMMENT

Michael X. Repka, MD

For guarded superior oblique tenotomies in Brown syndrome, I prefer a loop of suture rather than a silicone spacer, as it seems to present less bulk of material in the supranasal quadrant than scleral buckling silicone. I do not think that there is any effective force transmission through the scleral buckling material to the original insertion site beyond that afforded by the connective tissues surrounding the tendon of the superior oblique as it passes from the trochlea to below the superior rectus muscle. Both procedures make it easy to identify the cut ends of the tendon if necessary at a subsequent operation.

COMMENT

Marshall M. Parks, MD

The oblique muscles raise the challenge in understanding their pathology by an octave or more compared to the challenges offered by the rectus muscles. Their reputation established them as the last bastion of motility disorders to be conquered. Of the two, the superior oblique was billed early on as the chief offender. *Noli me tangere* ("do not touch me") was the label the superior oblique received just a century ago. Throughout the past half century, the unconquerable superior oblique has been tamed to the degree that it is now approachable. It has received more attention and research on all its details and with greater focus on surgical techniques than any of the other five extraocular muscles.

In 1949, Brown introduced the syndrome he speculated to be a shortened inelastic sheath of the anterior (reflected) component of the superior oblique tendon. It quickly became the newest *noli me tangere* in strabismology. All surgical attempts were unsuccessful at best and often disastrous. Berke's operation of a blind sweep of a muscle hook in the sub-Tenon's space to engage the superior oblique tendon and pull it forward into the operative field also ensnarled the Tenon's capsule, which was wrapped around the tendon and was erroneously described as the tendon sheath. The hook with its captured tendon was exposed by incising and tearing the Tenon's capsule before tenotomizing or tenectomizing it nasal to the superior rectus. The rent produced in Tenon's capsule allowed the extraconal fat to enter the sup-Tenon's space and adhere to the sclera, creating a superior oblique adherence (fat adherence) in the orbit, with the motility of the globe becoming worse than it was before surgery. Massive intraoperative hemorrhage, from the blind sweep tearing out the superior nasal vortex vein, and permanent ptosis were frequent complications.

Newer visualized approaches to the tendon have eliminated the complications associated with early surgical attempts. The almost invariable end result of a complete superior oblique tenotomy was a gradual superior oblique palsy, which then required surgery. The tight, inelastic shortened tendon must be lengthened, but the needed control of the tendon lengthening to the level that prevents paresis of the tendon is provided by the 6.0 mm Wright silicone spacer inserted between the cut ends, plus exquisite technique that preserves all the intermuscular tissue that enshrouds the reflected portion of the tendon. Brown syndrome no longer is a *noli me tangere*.

SUPERIOR OBLIQUE OVERACTION

Superior oblique overaction, characterized by excessive depression of the eye in the field of action of the superior oblique in comparison to the abducted/infraducted fellow eye, can be categorized as primary or secondary. Both are relatively rare compared to overaction of the inferior oblique.

Primary superior oblique overaction is relatively uncommon but does occur. It is always bilateral, although it can be asymmetric. Superior oblique overaction is more commonly secondary to either ipsilateral inferior oblique palsy or an infraduction deficiency in the opposite eye from either restriction or paresis. One of the most common reasons for down-gaze restriction resulting in apparent superior oblique overaction of the fellow eye is superior rectus restriction from long-standing superior oblique palsy.

Unilateral Overaction. Unilateral superior oblique overaction is invariably due to ipsilateral inferior oblique weakness or contralateral deficiency of infraduction secondary to restriction of down gaze or weakness of the inferior rectus (Fig. 3–12). Contralateral superior rectus restriction is discussed more fully later in the chapter. In general, weakening of the overacting superior oblique should be avoided when the overaction is due to contralateral superior rectus restriction. Instead, the tight superior rectus should be recessed.

COMMENT

Marshall M. Parks, MD

> Primary overaction of the ipsilateral superior oblique can masquerade as inferior oblique muscle palsy, except for the fact that the third step of the three-step test does not support this diagnosis.

Bilateral Overaction. Bilateral superior oblique overaction manifests as an overdepression of each adducted eye and is usually associated with a large A pattern. The eyes can be straight in the primary position, but there is usually an associated horizontal strabismus, either esotropia or exotropia.

Bilateral overaction is frequently, but not always, associated with subnormal binocular vision and sometimes other, more extensive central nervous system dis-

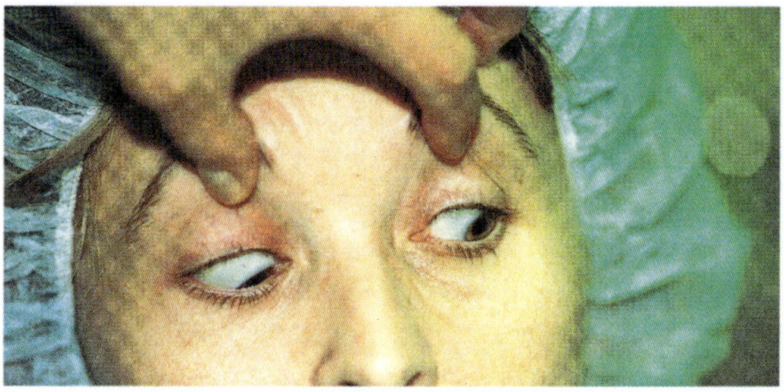

Figure 3–12. Superior oblique overaction secondary to restriction of down gaze in the opposite eye in long-standing large hyperdeviation from congenital left superior oblique palsy.

ease, including hydrocephalus, myelomeningocele, posterior fossa abnormalities, or periventricular leukomalacia. There is also a known triad of A-pattern exotropia with bilateral superior oblique overaction and dissociated vertical deviation (Fig. 3–13).

Surgical Treatment. Large A patterns with marked superior oblique overaction can be treated with bilateral superior oblique weakening. The author usually prefers bilateral superior oblique tenotomy, performed nasal to the superior rectus through a superior temporal incision. Superior oblique tenotomy in this setting tends to be self-grading. Other surgeons prefer a disinsertion of the superior oblique insertion, counting on the attachments to the overlying superior rectus to keep the superior oblique tendon from retracting far. This procedure is not as effective for weakening significantly overacting superior oblique muscles.

With this clinical entity, the risk of causing a symptomatic consecutive superior oblique palsy is very low, in contrast to superior oblique tenotomy for Brown syndrome. Most patients with marked superior oblique overaction and an A pattern have no or only gross stereopsis, which explains why they rarely experience postoperative diplopia. For these reasons, the author does not consider any benefits of placing a silicone spacer to outweigh the added effort and potential complications associated with its placement in cases of bilateral primary superior oblique overaction.

WARNING

If a patient has high-grade stereopsis (more than 60 seconds arc), bilateral superior oblique weakening must be done with great caution, if at all, because of the substantial risk of producing postoperative torsional diplopia.

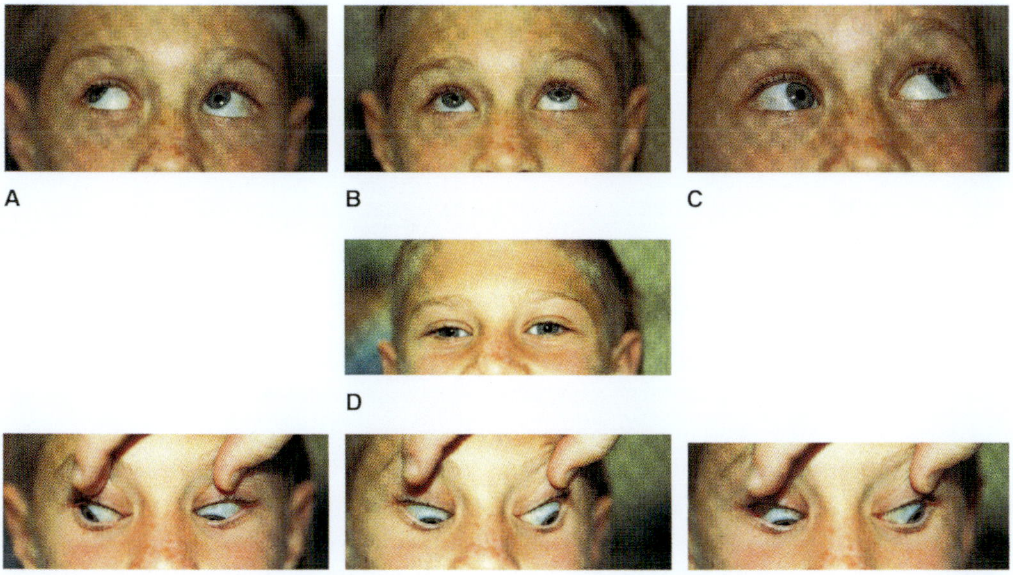

A B C D E F G

Figure 3–13A–G. Triad of A-pattern exotropia with superior oblique overaction and dissociated vertical deviation.

COMMENT

M. Edward Wilson, MD

The warning against performing superior oblique tendon tenotomy bilaterally in patients with high-grade stereopsis is justified, but not for the reason given. A tenotomy of truly overacting superior obliques would be unlikely to produce enough extorsion to cause torsional diplopia. The more likely danger is a slightly asymmetric result, with a small vertical deviation in the primary position resulting in a head tilt postoperatively. Patients with monofixation syndrome (absence of high-grade stereopsis) are more tolerant of these small hypertropias and do not usually show a head tilt postoperatively.

COMMENT

Marshall M. Parks, MD

It is in treating the patient with bilateral overacting superior obliques and A-pattern exotropia that the author has directed a warning against superior oblique surgery if the stereoacuity is excellent, which means that the patient is a bifixator as opposed to a monofixator. The bifixating patient with A-pattern exodeviation has difficulty controlling eye alignment in down gaze, causing near-vision symptoms with sustained reading and like activities from the increased exodeviation and incyclophoria in that eye position.

Bilateral superior oblique weakening associated with some exodeviation corrective surgery seems reasonable, but the postoperative incyclodiplopia in the primary position is most displeasing for the patient. For the bifixating patient it is intolerable, but the monofixator is less bothered. Prisms are unable to bring relief. Lowering the chin while keeping the eyes elevated reduces the incyclodiplopia. However, the symptoms are more severe for the bifixator. Those who have only extramacular binocular vision and no macular binocular vision tolerate the symptoms much better. Stereoacuity measured preoperatively is the most dependable assessment to use for determining whether the patient is a bifixator and should not have the superior oblique tenotomized.

SUPERIOR OBLIQUE UNDERACTION, OR PALSY

Underaction of the superior oblique can be seen with marked inferior oblique overaction, such as in the congenital esotropia complex, but this diagnosis should be apparent by the clinical history and setting. The underaction will typically normalize following appropriate weakening of the inferior obliques. It can also be associated with congenital laxity of the superior oblique tendons or with rotated orbits, causing upward displacement of the medial rectus muscles/pulleys, in which case superior oblique tucks or vertical shifts of the horizontal rectus muscles, respectively, may be indicated. In general, superior oblique underaction is more commonly termed *superior oblique palsy*.

Superior oblique palsy is the most commonly occurring cyclovertical muscle palsy. Approximately three-quarters of these cases are congenital and one-quarter are due to identifiable acquired causes. These figures differ widely among practitioners, depending on referral patterns.

Congenital Fourth Nerve Palsy, or Superior Oblique Paresis. Most superior oblique palsies are congenital and unilateral. The palsy may present in infancy with torticollis, usually on the side opposite the palsy. Less severe congenital palsies may present later in childhood or even well into adulthood with torticollis, diplopia, or asthenopia.

The majority of congenital superior oblique palsies are associated with laxity of the involved superior oblique tendon, as determined by intraoperative traction testing. The significance of this tendon laxity is clear: it is of great importance in formulating a surgical treatment plan. The cause of the laxity is much less clear. Is the laxity a primary anatomic abnormality of the structure of the superior oblique tendon complex? Is the laxity secondary to a denervation atrophy? The answers to these questions are unknown, but some clues are available.

Denervation atrophy of the skeletal muscle portion of the superior oblique, as diagnosed by cross-sectional CT or magnetic resonance imaging (MRI) scan, may be present in both congenital and acquired cases (Fig. 3–14). Other cases of congenital palsy in children have been associated with little or no difference in cross-sectional area between the palsied and the normal side.

It may be that some congenitally lax superior oblique tendons represent the opposite end of the clinical spectrum of superior oblique tendon abnormality from the tight tendons found in varying degrees in Brown syndrome. The ultimate anatomic abnormality of the superior oblique—complete absence—is a well-known but rare cause of congenital superior oblique palsy.

Acquired Palsy. Acquired neurogenic superior oblique palsy is due to injury to the trochlear nerve anywhere along its path from the dorsal midbrain, along the tentorium cerebelli, through the cavernous sinus, and into the orbit. This long course makes this nerve particularly susceptible to trauma, which is the most common cause of acquired superior oblique palsy. The trauma is frequently severe closed-head injury but can be direct trauma to the trochlea–tendon complex, including iatrogenic trauma from sinus, orbital, or neurologic surgery. A significant blow to the head, resulting in loss of consciousness, is typically required to cause superior oblique palsy; a palsy diagnosed following less severe head injury should prompt a search for another cause. Other potential causes include vascular malformation or infarction, inflammation, infection, tumor, neuromuscular disorder (such as myasthenia gravis), iatrogenic causes, or previously unnoticed congenital palsy.

Signs and Symptoms. Since the superior oblique principally depresses and intorts the eye, palsy of this muscle will result in varying degrees of hypertropia and excyclotorsion. In general, congenital palsies tend to be associated with greater ver-

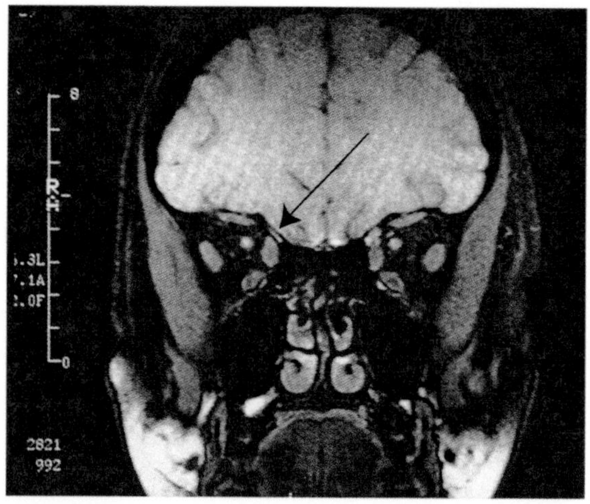

A

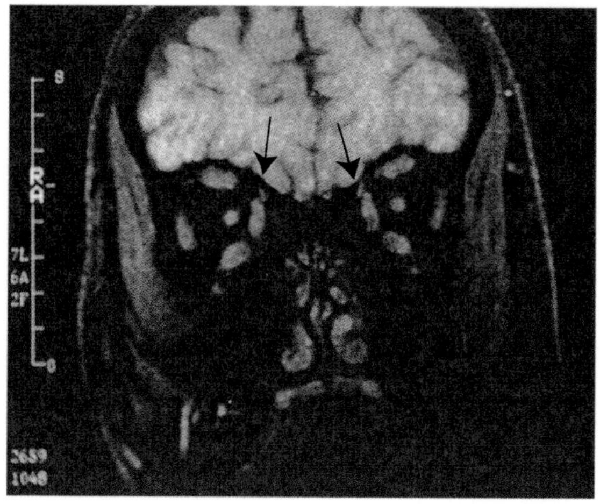

B

Figure 3–14. Unilateral and bilateral superior oblique palsy. (*A*) Cross-sectional magnetic resonance imaging scan showing atrophy of the skeletal muscle portion of the affected superior oblique in unilateral superior oblique palsy. (*B*) Bilateral denervation atrophy of superior obliques in acquired (traumatic) bilateral superior oblique palsy.

tical deviations and little or no excyclotorsion, the latter perhaps due to sensorial adaptations in early childhood. Acquired palsies frequently have smaller deviations and relatively larger degrees of torsion. However, there is enough overlap that neither the magnitude of deviation nor the degree of subjective excyclotorsion can be used to differentiate between congenital and acquired palsies. If greater than 10° of excyclotorsion is measured, a bilateral palsy should be suspected.

A compensatory head posture is the most common presenting sign of superior oblique palsy (Fig. 3–15). The torticollis is typically away from the side of the lesion to promote fusion, but in rare instances, the head tilt is toward the affected side to maximally separate the diplopic images.

A frequently overlooked but important clinical sign is the characteristic facial asymmetry that occurs in patients with torticollis from a young age. This facial asymmetry is due to a midfacial hypoplasia and is recognized by a shallowing of the midface between the lateral canthus and the corner of the mouth. This asym-

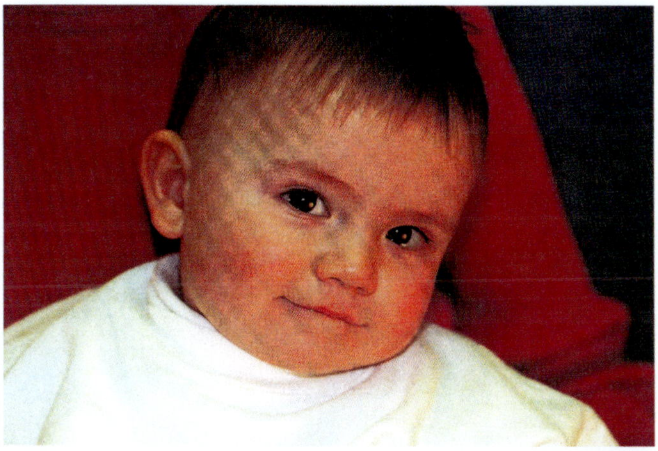

A

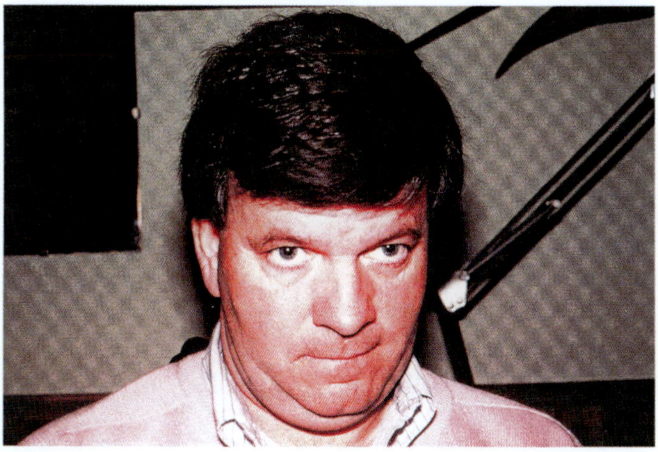

B

Figure 3–15. Superior oblique palsy in an infant and an adult. (*A*) Typical appearance of an infant with torticollis secondary to congenital right superior oblique palsy. (*B*) Typical chin-down position of an adult with acquired bilateral superior oblique palsy.

metry always develops on the dependent side of the face (the lower side), regardless of which side the palsy is on.

Facial asymmetry, while characteristic of congenital superior oblique palsy, is not specific for it. It can occur with any cause of torticollis in infancy, including congenital muscular torticollis and the Klippel-Feil anomaly. However, this important finding in an older patient with superior oblique palsy can obviate the need for an expensive and unnecessary neurologic workup, since the facial asymmetry suggests a congenital cause (Fig. 3–16).

This midfacial hypoplasia should not be confused with plagiocephaly caused by coronal synostosis. In these cases of skull asymmetry with which there is an associated superior oblique palsy, the palsy is very likely caused by the relative displacement of the trochlea due to the premature suture closure.

Bilateral acquired superior oblique palsy is typified by a large degree of excyclotorsion, a small primary-position deviation, and a V pattern, with increasing esotropia in down gaze. Alternating head tilt (left hypertropia on left head tilt and

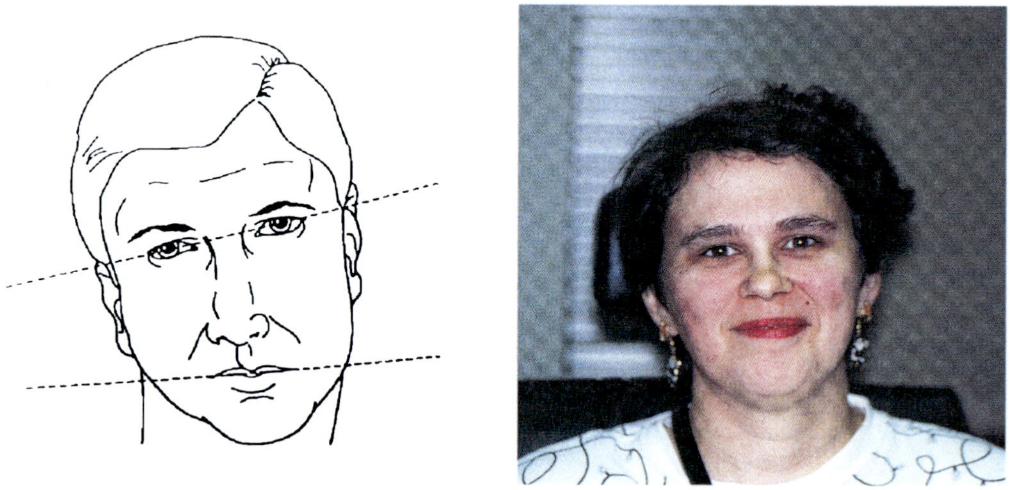

Figure 3–16. Typical facial asymmetry. Note the midfacial hypoplasia with decreased distance between the lateral canthus and the corner of the mouth on the smaller side. Imaginary horizontal lines drawn through the lateral canthus of each eye and through the corners of the mouth will intersect in the space on the side of facial hypoplasia.

right hypertropia on right head tilt) is diagnostic. However, in some cases, the vertical deviation decreases to zero rather than shifting to the opposite hypertropia, suggesting a unilateral palsy. This condition sometimes becomes known as a *masked bilateral palsy*, with the bilaterality becoming apparent only after the first (more obvious) side has been treated surgically.

Diagnosis.

Three-step test. The diagnosis is suggested by the findings on the three-step test, which is applicable to any unoperated patient with an isolated cyclovertical muscle palsy (Fig. 3–17). In this case, the patient will have a hypertropia that increases on gaze away from the side of the lesion and increases on head tilt toward the side of the lesion. For example, a right superior oblique palsy will typically have a right hypertropia that increases on left gaze and right head tilt. It must be borne in mind that the three-step test identifies the palsied muscle in cases of isolated cyclovertical muscle palsy only; it is not applicable to other causes of hypertropia, such as blowout fracture, thyroid ophthalmopathy, dissociated vertical deviation, monocular elevation deficiency, Brown syndrome, or any other restrictive or innervational abnormality.

Torsion. Subjective torsion should be measured with the double Maddox rod in any patient capable of performing this test. Torsion can also be assessed, though less precisely, with indirect ophthalmoscopy of the fundus or fundus photography. A few helpful generalizations regarding torsion findings are as follows:

1. Congenital superior oblique palsy, as a rule, has little or no measurable objective or subjective torsion.

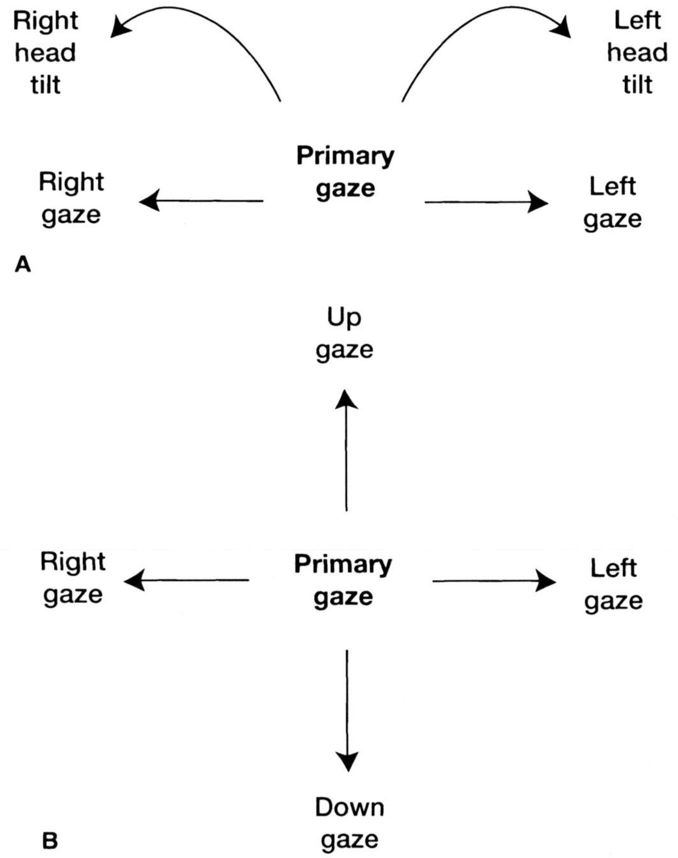

Figure 3–17. Three-step test. (*A*) Positions of gaze required for diagnosis of superior oblique palsy. (*B*) Positions of gaze required for making a surgical plan for superior oblique palsy.

2. Acquired superior oblique palsy is usually associated with measurable excyclotorsion.
3. Large degrees of torsion (greater than 10°), which are frequently accompanied by spontaneous complaints of torsional diplopia, suggest a bilateral palsy.

Versions. Three abnormalities in versions should be searched for:

1. *Inferior oblique overaction* (Fig. 3–18A): Inferior oblique overaction is common and is present to some degree in almost all cases of superior oblique palsy. It may be subtle or even negligible in some acquired cases, especially in elderly patients.
2. *Superior oblique underaction* (Fig. 3–18B): Significant superior oblique underaction is frequently not manifest in cases of superior oblique palsy. Marked underaction of the superior oblique suggests an anatomic abnormality, such as excessive tendon laxity or, in extreme cases, absence of the tendon.
3. *Contralateral superior oblique overaction* (Fig. 3–18C): This apparent superior oblique overaction in the opposite eye is secondary to restriction of

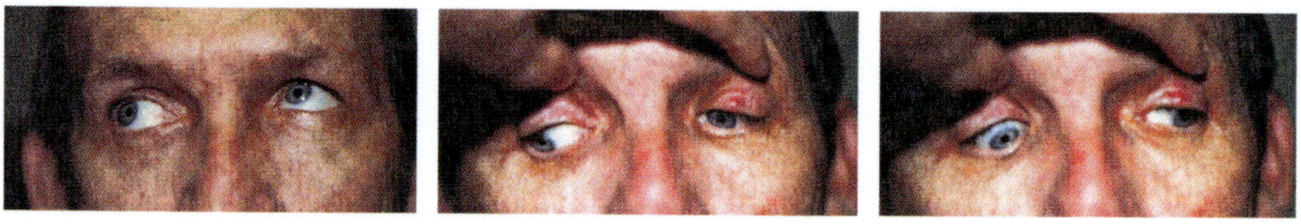

A B C

Figure 3–18. Adult with congenital superior oblique palsy showing all three common version abnormalities. (*A*) Inferior oblique overaction (left). (*B*) Superior oblique underaction (left). (*C*) Contralateral (right) superior oblique overaction secondary to ipsilateral (left) superior rectus restriction.

down gaze in abduction of the palsied side from contracture of the ipsilateral superior rectus. This occurs only in long-standing, large hyperdeviation. Treatment requires recession of the affected superior rectus, *not* weakening of the contralateral superior oblique.

Surgical Treatment. Asymptomatic mild palsies can be observed or ignored until they become symptomatic or manifest with a compensatory head tilt. Small, relatively comitant deviations, especially those occurring in the elderly, may benefit from treatment with prisms. Most cases of superior oblique palsy presenting to the strabismologist will require surgical attention.

Surgical principles. The principle of matching the field(s) of greatest deviation to the muscles whose greatest action is in those fields is credited to the landmark contribution of Knapp in his classification of superior oblique palsy. Although some of the specific treatment recommendations from that classification are no longer considered optimal, the importance of the general principle remains. To this treatment scaffold can be added information derived from observations of deviation magnitude, superior rectus contracture, superior oblique laxity, and torsion to come up with a logical treatment plan for each patient.

The five pieces of information needed to formulate the surgical treatment plan for a patient with unilateral superior oblique palsy are as follows:

1. Magnitude (alternate cover testing) of deviation in primary position and left, right, up, and down gazes
2. Assessment of versions
3. Measurement of torsion
4. Presence of superior rectus contracture
5. Assessment of superior oblique tendon laxity

The first four have already been discussed. The last, tendon laxity, is diagnosed by intraoperative superior oblique traction testing.

Traction test. Intraoperative traction testing of the superior oblique has become an indispensable part of evaluating patients with superior oblique palsy. It is especially relevant for young children in whom precise motility measurements cannot be obtained. Traction testing identifies very lax tendons that should be tucked and, just as important, identifies tendons of normal length that should not be tucked because of the risk of causing Brown syndrome. Even though the majority of superior oblique tendons in congenital palsy have some degree of excess laxity, most do not have the marked laxity that requires a tuck.

The technique for assessing laxity of the superior oblique tendon is based on the method of *exaggerated forced ductions* of the obliques described by Guyton for evaluating patients with superior oblique overaction. It has been modified to help emphasize the laxity in these redundant tendons. The four steps are as follows (Fig. 3–19):

1. With the surgeon seated above the head of the supine anesthetized patient, two toothed forceps are used to grasp the limbus diagonally, that is, at the 2 and 8 o'clock positions on the left eye and at the 4 and 10 o'clock positions on the right eye.
2. The eye is rotated up into an elevated, adducted position in the superonasal quadrant while the globe is simultaneously pushed down toward the orbital apex. This maneuver puts the reflected tendon on maximal stretch, thereby showing the degree of laxity between the tendon's firm attachments to the trochlea and its insertion onto the globe.
3. Once the tendon is put on stretch, the eye is moved back and forth (temporally and nasally) while the tendon is kept taut. This back-and-forth movement allows the surgeon to *feel* the tendon as a band across which the globe is rocked.
4. Steps 1 to 3 are repeated on the fellow eye.

Important points regarding the traction test are summarized here. All normal superior oblique tendons can be easily felt using this technique. Becoming comfortable using the method on normal patients will allow the surgeon to be more aware of what an abnormal tendon feels like. Because there is a range of normal tendon laxity, it is the *relative* laxity of the tendon compared with that of its fellow eye that is the determining factor. A subjective grading scale is used to compare the paretic and normal tendons.

1− Tendon is only mildly lax.
2− Tendon is obviously more lax than normal.
3− Tendon is markedly lax but definitely present.
4− Tendon cannot be felt with certainty. The tendon may be absent, but some tendons are so lax that the end point of the test comes from resistance of other tissues attached to the globe, not from the outstretched tendon itself.

In general, 4− tendons should always be tucked; 3− tendons are usually tucked, 2− tendons are rarely tucked, and 1− tendons are almost never tucked. The gain from tucking 1− and 2− tendons usually is not outweighed by the potential risk of causing Brown syndrome.

The vigorous traction-testing maneuver will easily tear the fragile conjunctiva of adults. It is generally more valuable in children; if it is done in older adults, locking toothed forceps should be used on the episclera and sclera, not just on the conjunctiva.

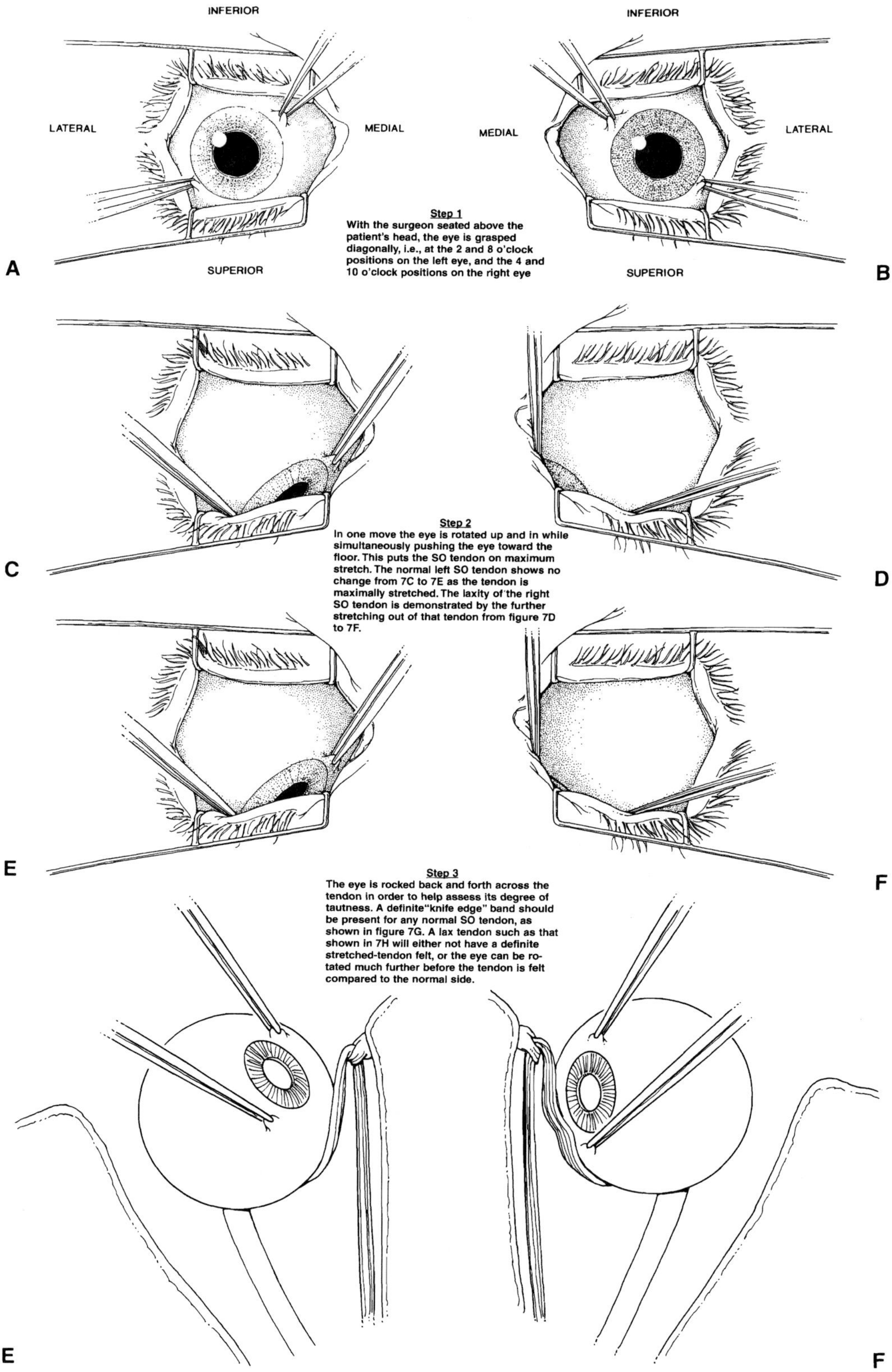

Figure 3–19A–H. Traction test (see text for explanation of steps). (Redrawn from Plager DA: Superior oblique palsy and superior oblique myokymia. In: Rosenbaum AL, Santiago AP, eds: *Clinical Strabismus Management: Principles and Surgical Techniques*. Philadelphia: WB Saunders Co; 1999, 224–225, Figure 15–7A–H. Copyright 1999, with permission from Elsevier. 219–229, copyright 1999, with permission from Elsevier.)

Treatment algorithm. A suggested treatment algorithm follows. It does not cover all permutations of deviation that may present, but it can serve as a useful framework that is applicable to a large number of patients with this diagnosis.

If the patient has a deviation of less than 15Δ in the primary position, one-muscle surgery is probably sufficient. The choice of which muscle to operate on depends on evaluation of the inferior oblique:

1. If there is inferior oblique overaction, the muscle is weakened by either myectomy or graded recession, depending on the surgeon's preference. It is rare to overcorrect a patient with superior oblique palsy and inferior oblique overaction by weakening the ipsilateral inferior oblique. The only question is whether that procedure alone is sufficient to correct the deviation.
2. If there is no inferior oblique overaction, the following alternatives exist:
   (a) If the ipsilateral superior rectus is restricted, the superior rectus is recessed. As with any form of strabismus, it is desirable to relieve any restriction that is present. However, significant superior rectus restriction is unlikely in patients with small deviations.
   (b) If there is marked laxity of the superior oblique, the tendon is tucked. Marked superior oblique laxity is rarely encountered in patients without inferior oblique overaction. Therefore, in most cases of small deviation with no inferior oblique overaction, the most logical choice will be the following:
   (c) The contralateral inferior rectus is recessed.

If the primary-position deviation is greater than 15Δ, surgery on two or more muscles may be necessary to correct it. It cannot be overemphasized that if there is doubt as to whether a second muscle needs to be operated on, the surgeon should always err on the side of less surgery. Undercorrecting patients who have built up relatively large vertical fusional amplitudes in that direction is far preferable to even a small overcorrection, which will cause symptoms (including diplopia) that may be worse than those present preoperatively.

If surgery on a second muscle is deemed necessary, it can be chosen based on the following alternatives:

1. Ipsilateral superior rectus recession if this muscle is restricted
2. Ipsilateral superior oblique tuck if there is marked laxity of the tendon
3. Contralateral inferior rectus recession

A combination of these choices can be used if the deviation is so large (greater than 30Δ in primary position) that three muscles need to be operated.

WARNING

In cases of apparent contralateral superior oblique overaction, a tenotomy or other weakening procedure should *never* be performed on the offending superior oblique; instead, the ipsilateral superior rectus should be recessed. Weakening the contralateral superior oblique in a case of unilateral superior oblique palsy will result in an iatrogenic bilateral superior oblique palsy that is very difficult to correct.

The author no longer does superior oblique tucks, except in those patients who definitely need them to correct their strabismus—patients with excessive laxity of the involved tendon. In all other patients, the misalignment can be corrected with some combination of weakening procedures on other muscles of one or both eyes, as described above, which can be done without the significant risk of causing a Brown syndrome. The exception is the large torsion that can be present in bilateral acquired palsy and requires a procedure aimed at the torsion, such as a Harada-Ito procedure, as discussed further in the section "Bilateral Acquired Palsy."

COMMENT

Edward G. Buckley, MD

While I generally agree with the surgical recommendations given, it is important to know that deviations greater than 15Δ can be treated effectively with one-muscle surgery, either a superior oblique tuck or an inferior oblique myectomy/recession. I have treated large primary deviations of up to 30Δ with one inferior oblique recession. In those circumstances, the entire primary deviation was eliminated and a small residual hyperdeviation on lateral gaze persisted. Over the ensuing 12 to 24 months, this deviation effectively disappeared as well. Every effort must be made not to overcorrect a superior oblique palsy.

A combination of a superior oblique tuck and an ipsilateral inferior oblique recession must be used with caution since this will often create an overcorrection on lateral gaze that will be quite bothersome to the patient. If two-muscle surgery is considered, I prefer to operate on both eyes since the inferior rectus recession can be graded more precisely and the risks of overcorrection minimized. In adult patients with large deviations, I favor ipsilateral inferior oblique myectomy and contralateral inferior rectus recession on adjustable sutures. In patients with significant underaction of the superior oblique with large deviations on down and lateral gazes, a combination superior oblique tuck and contralateral inferior rectus recession on adjustable suture can be very effective.

Young children. In infants and toddlers with torticollis due to superior oblique palsy, it is not possible to obtain motility measurements in different gaze fields. This has caused some ophthalmologists to delay surgery for years until precise measurements can be made. Delay is unwise because progressive loss of fusion is possible and there are potential adverse effects on the child's facial development.

Theoretically, development of facial asymmetry should be preventable by early surgery to correct the torticollis. This supposition has been borne out in many children with congenital superior oblique palsy who were operated on at a young age. If the head posture is surgically corrected before facial asymmetry is apparent, it does not develop later.

The failure rate when correcting torticollis in infants with superior oblique palsy is high after inferior oblique weakening alone. In this situation, use of the intraoperative traction test of superior oblique laxity is especially helpful. If the tendon is markedly lax, as it usually is in infants with torticollis, a superior oblique tuck should be performed in addition to the inferior oblique weakening. If the superior oblique is not significantly lax, only the inferior oblique should be operated on.

The surgeon cannot determine preoperatively how many millimeters of tendon should be tucked. An intraoperative assessment of tendon laxity is required. The end point of the tuck is a feel on traction testing that is the same as that on the normal side. It is not necessary to create a Brown syndrome to achieve an effect if the ipsilateral inferior oblique is weakened at the same time.

The presence of a horizontal deviation or amblyopia in patients with congenital superior oblique palsy should alert the surgeon that the superior oblique tendon may be absent. The traction test can prove noninvasively that the tendon is present. However, if the test suggests that the tendon may be absent, surgical exploration is necessary for confirmation. Occasionally, a superior oblique tendon is so lax that it cannot be appreciated by the traction test. If the tendon is absent, the author empirically recesses the ipsilateral superior rectus by a moderate amount, in addition to performing inferior oblique weakening as the first procedure.

COMMENT

Marshall M. Parks, MD

The author's discussion about young children or infants with torticollis secondary to unilateral congenital superior oblique palsy brings to the attention of the ophthalmologist all the correct facts and advice for therapy. But I wish to emphasize the need to treat the torticollis early and correctly: *early* means in the first several months of age, and *correctly*, in large part, involves the choice of the particular muscle to be selected for the first surgery. For older children and adults, I find it ideal to operate on the ipsilateral antagonist or the yoke, rather than strengthening the palsied muscle with avoided Brown syndrome. But this plan has proved inadequate to overcome the torticollis in infants compared to the tuck of the superior oblique.

In observing patients who did not receive expeditious and timely surgery to correct the torticollis, one is struck by the impairment of their looks by an asymmetric face. Older patients complain of neck pain resulting from cervical arthritis. It is obvious from these observations that the pediatric ophthalmologist should take a page from the pediatric orthopedist's book. Only the pediatric ophthalmologist can prevent the asymmetric facial blemish and the neck agony in adulthood. The orthopedist is very aware of the permanent harm that results from delaying infantile torticollis correction. The ophthalmologist is more focused on correcting misaligned eyes and delaying therapy until patients are older, when a better examination may provide more reliable information. The ophthalmologist must adjust the priorities in the treatment of the child with torticollis; it is most important to straighten the head as early as possible.

Bilateral acquired palsy. Surgical treatment is aimed at reducing the large degree of torsion, nullifying the primary-position hypertropia, collapsing the V pattern, and reducing any chin-down head posture. Bilateral inferior oblique weakening is usually insufficient to correct this problem and is not a good first-choice procedure. More effective is weakening the yoke muscle (contralateral inferior rectus of each palsied superior oblique). The recession is empirically moderate (5.0 to 6.0 mm) for a symmetric palsy and no primary-position deviation but can be modified to adjust for any primary-position deviation. For instance, a patient with bilateral superior oblique palsy and 5Δ of left hypertropia in the primary position might benefit from a right inferior rectus recession of 6.0 mm and a left inferior rectus recession of 4.0 mm. This will help correct any V pattern, but it is not sufficient to correct large degrees of excyclotorsion.

Large amounts of excyclotorsion (more than 10°) require a procedure aimed specifically at reducing it. Bilateral inferior oblique weakening is not sufficient. Harada and Ito described splitting the superior oblique and advancing the anterior half of the tendon. The anterior fibers are primarily responsible for the torsional action of the superior oblique. The primarily vertically acting posterior fibers are left undisturbed. A modification of the Harada-Ito procedure advances the anterior superior oblique fibers to the superior border of the lateral rectus 8.0 mm posterior to the lateral rectus insertion. Use of an adjustable procedure has also been described.

COMMENT
Michael X. Repka, MD

I have found that the Harada-Ito procedure tends to lose its effectiveness over time and that adherence of the tendon fibers to the surface of the globe is sufficiently secure when performed with nonabsorbable sutures. I perform any adjustment in the operating room, monitoring the fundus torsion. Almost all of these procedures initially appear to have overcorrected the extorsion, but this finding rapidly disappears.

COMMENT
Gunter K. von Noorden, MD

My indications for a Harada-Ito procedure differ somewhat from those of the author. The only indication I know of is an isolated, acquired, symptomatic excyclotropia as the only presenting sign of a very mild superior oblique paresis without a vertical strabismus component. Correction of the vertical deviation in patients with trochlear palsy by strengthening the action of the superior oblique and weakening the action of the inferior oblique suffices, as a rule, to correct the accompanying excyclotropia as well.

Incidentally, such patients respond equally well to nasal transposition of the inferior rectus muscle of the affected eye, a procedure I prefer over the Harada-Ito operation when the excyclotropia is limited to down gaze.

The medial rectus muscles can be transposed down one-half to a full tendon width to correct the V pattern, and this may be combined with a recession if there is more than 15Δ of esotropia in primary gaze.

COMMENT

Edward G. Buckley, MD

In patients with bilateral superior oblique palsy, strengthening the superior oblique muscles is almost always necessary. These muscles are grossly underacting, and recession of the inferior rectus muscle does not usually, by itself, result in a satisfactory outcome. I prefer superior oblique tucks to the Harada-Ito procedure, since significant excyclotorsion exists on down gaze, as well as a duction deficit in most of these patients. The Harada-Ito procedure can be effective for the torsion, but it does not provide as much depression as is usually needed. For small deviations, it is fine. If a significant esotropia exists on down gaze, then medial rectus recessions with infraplacement are often necessary since the A pattern created by superior oblique tucks or inferior rectus recessions is usually not significant enough to eliminate the down-gaze esotropia. In my experience, in very mild bilateral superior oblique palsies, bilateral inferior rectus recessions will suffice. All other situations require bilateral superior oblique tucks in combination with inferior rectus recessions and medial rectus recessions.

COMMENT

Marshall M. Parks, MD

In bilateral acquired superior oblique palsy, the dominant deviation problem for the patient is excyclotropia. In unilateral cases, there is a larger vertical deviation with minimal cyclodeviation. But the more the bilateral superior oblique palsy manifests symmetric involvement in each eye, the more the strabismic deviation is manifest as a cyclodeviation, which is additive from each eye, while the vertical deviation in one eye cancels that in the other eye, tending to nullify the vertical component. The V-pattern esotropia is also apparent due to the diminished secondary abduction function maximally provided by the superior obliques, allowing the tone in the inferior rectus muscles to produce the esodeviation in down gaze. It is fortunate that the Harada-Ito operation could be devised to correct for all three deviations.

Lastly, a comment on Bielschowsky and how he influenced our knowledge about the cyclovertical muscles. His knowledge about the basic functions and physiology of these muscles laid the foundation for practically all advances in the techniques for managing the strabismic disorders affecting these muscles. Prior to Bielschowsky, the diagnosis of oblique muscle palsies and overaction was rare. Far more superior oblique palsies were misdiagnosed as superior rectus palsies. In the early twentieth century, superior rectus palsy was declared to be the most common cause of torticollis. With such ignorance, one can easily understand why there was a dictum to not touch the superior oblique muscle.

ACKNOWLEDGMENT
Some material on superior oblique palsy in this chapter has been reproduced from Plager DA: Superior oblique palsy and superior oblique myokymia. In: Rosenbaum AL, Santiago AP, eds: *Clinical Strabismus Management: Principles and Surgical Techniques*. Philadelphia: WB Saunders Co; 1999, 219–229. Copyright 1999, with permission from Elsevier.

Suggested Readings

Brown HW: Congenital structural muscle anomalies. In: Allen JH, ed: *Symposium on Strabismus: Transactions of the New Orleans Academy of Ophthalmology*. St Louis: CV Mosby Co; 1950, 205–236.

Helveston EM: *Surgical Management of Strabismus: An Atlas of Strabismus Surgery*, 4th ed. St Louis: CV Mosby Co; 1993.

Helveston EM, Mora JS, Lipsky SN, et al: Surgical treatment of superior oblique palsy. *Trans Am Ophthalmol Soc* 1996; 94:315–328; discussion 328–334.

Knapp P: Classification and treatment of superior oblique palsy. *Am Orthopt J* 1974; 24:18–22.

Mitchell PR, Parks MM: Surgery of bilateral superior oblique palsy. *Ophthalmology* 1982; 89:484–488.

Parks MM: Isolated cyclovertical muscle palsy. *Arch Ophthalmol* 1958; 60:1027–1035.

Paysee EA, Coats DK, Plager DA: Facial asymmetry and tendon laxity in superior oblique palsy. *J Pediatr Ophthalmol Strabismus* 1995; 32:158–161.

Plager DA: Tendon laxity in superior oblique palsy. *Ophthalmology* 1992; 99:1032–1038.

Plager DA: Superior oblique palsy and superior oblique myokymia. In: Rosenbaum AL, Santiago AP, eds: *Clinical Strabismus Management: Principles and Surgical Techniques*. Philadelphia: WB Saunders Co; 1999, 219–229.

Pollard ZF: Inferior oblique paresis: a benign entity. *Ann Ophthalmol* 1986; 18:178–180.

Rosenbaum AL, Santiago AP, eds: *Clinical Strabismus Management: Principles and Surgical Techniques*. Philadelphia: WB Saunders Co; 1999.

von Noorden GK: *Binocular Vision and Ocular Motility: Theory and Management of Strabismus*, 5th ed. St Louis; CV Mosby Co; 1996.

Wilson ME, Eustis HS Jr, Parks MM: Brown's syndrome. *Surv Ophthalmol* 1989; 34:153–172.

Wright KW: Superior oblique silicone expander for Brown syndrome and superior oblique overaction. *J Pediatr Ophthalmol Strabismus* 1991; 28:101–107.

4

Dissociated Deviations

M. EDWARD WILSON

Dissociated strabismus, although common, is poorly understood. The classic pattern of the dissociated strabismus complex (DSC) is of a nonfixating eye slowly elevating, extorting, and abducting upon the spontaneous loss of binocular function or with cover testing (Fig. 4–1). A reversal of these movements is seen with recovery and refixation. Latent nystagmus is also usually present. Macular binocular vision is characteristically absent, and a history of infantile horizontal strabismus (congenital esotropia) is often present.

Included in DSC are movements in the vertical, horizontal, and torsional axes. Each component of the complex should be documented separately. Latent nystagmus should be included as part of the complex. Dissociated vertical deviation (DVD) and dissociated horizontal deviation (DHD), when manifest frequently, require separate surgical strategies but often are treated surgically together. True hypertropia, hypotropia, esotropia, or exotropia can coexist with DSC. Treatment plans must be individualized for these patients, addressing both the DSC and any coexisting horizontal or vertical tropia. Although recent theories of causation are fascinating, DSC will apparently remain an enigma for years to come.

TERMINOLOGY OF DISSOCIATED STRABISMUS COMPLEX

The many descriptive titles under which this strabismus complex has been reported over the past century attest to our incomplete understanding and characterization of its varied manifestations. *Dissociated vertical deviation*, attributed to Raab, became a commonly used label for this type of strabismus in the 1970s and 1980s. However, this label implies a purely vertical deviation. While it is well known that

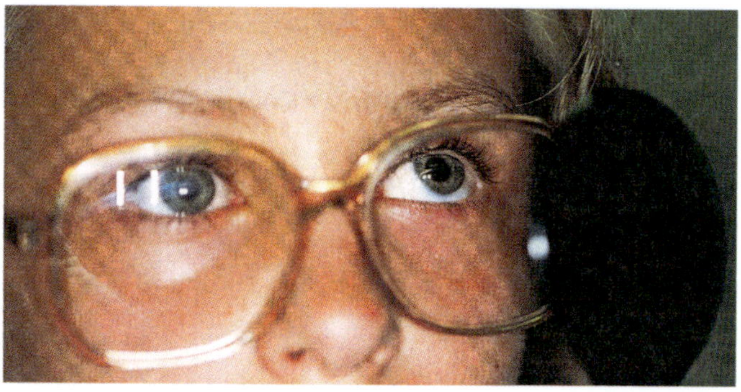

Figure 4–1. Dissociated strabismus complex shown during cover testing on the left eye. Behind the cover, the left eye is elevated, extorted, and abducted. This child had a history of surgically corrected congenital esotropia. She now has accommodative esotropia with coexistent bilateral DSC.

the slow elevation of the nonfixating eye is the most recognizable feature of dissociated strabismus, torsional or abducting components are usually also present and can predominate in one or both eyes, producing considerable diagnostic confusion. The term *dissociated strabismus complex* became more commonly used in the 1990s to describe the entire complex. It avoids the awkward semantics of describing dissociated strabismus manifesting almost entirely horizontal or torsional movements as a DVD.

Dissociated strabismus complex can be subdivided into *dissociated vertical deviation* (DVD), *dissociated horizontal deviation* (DHD), and *dissociated torsional deviation* (DTD) when recording patient examination findings. For instance, one eye may elevate markedly under cover with moderate extorsion and no visible abduction (4+ DVD, 3+ DTD), while the fellow eye may reveal marked abduction and mild extorsion but no visible elevation (4+ DHD, 2+ DTD) when covered. With this scheme, the familiar term *DVD* is still used to describe the vertical component of the complex. Because DHD has become a more clinically recognized entity, using *DSC* as an umbrella term avoids the temptation to overlook the intimate relationship between DVD, DHD, DTD, and latent nystagmus. If DVD or DHD is seen alone, it can still be labeled as such. On close observation, however, at least one other component of the complex is almost always present. In a patient with prominent DVD, documenting subtle coexisting DTD, DHD, or latent nystagmus gives the examiner more confidence in the diagnosis of dissociated strabismus and further justifies the DSC label.

THEORIES OF CAUSATION

The exact cause of DSC remains unknown. Helveston, in 1980, reviewed the literature on 10 different theories of the cause of DSC. The most important early work noted was done by Bielschowsky, who believed that DVD was due to alternating or intermittent excitations of both cerebral centers for vertical divergence. These centers, however, have never been found. Helveston supported and expanded on Bielschowsky's theory that DSC resulted from some maldeveloped supranuclear centers.

It is known that, phylogenetically, lower animals have both vertical and horizontal vergence centers. In humans, the development of high-grade fusion takes precedence and impedes the development of the vergence centers and thus the capacity for vertical and horizontal divergence. However, in the absence of adequate stimuli for fusion, the presence of functioning vestigial centers could result in DVD when the vertical vergence center is stimulated and in DHD when the horizontal vergence center is stimulated.

Past luminaries such as Brown, Scobee, and Verhoeff each concluded that a hypofunctioning superior oblique muscle could explain the vertical, torsional and horizontal movements seen in DSC. Cases of A-pattern exotropia, superior oblique muscle overaction, and DVD occurring simultaneously seemed to argue against superior oblique hypofunctioning as the cause of DVD. Perhaps it is possible for superior oblique muscle overaction to be manifest when the infranuclear pathways are functioning, and yet a hypofunctioning superior oblique muscle movement could occur when supernuclear pathways predominate.

In 1992, Enright recognized for the first time an association between vertical vergence and cycloversion. He observed that the vertical vergence producing a left hyperdeviation was associated with levocycloversion and vice versa. He calculated that the ratio between the vertical vergence and cycloversion was such that this cycloversion is likely mediated by the oblique muscles. The rectus muscles, if they contributed at all, functioned to counteract slightly the cycloversion that was noted. Enright concluded that the oblique muscles are the primary effectors of the vertical fusional reflex.

Van Rijn and Collewijn repeated the experiments of Enright, using search coil techniques for measuring eye movements. They confirmed the existence of the association between vertical vergence and cycloversion but disputed the role of the superior oblique muscles. These investigators concluded that the observed association between vertical vergence and cycloversion has a central origin and most likely results in the close association between the control of vertical and torsional movements at a central level. Therefore, these findings contradict the conclusion of Enright.

More recently, van Rijn et al. argued that disparity-induced vertical vergence and DVD share common neuronal pathways because of similar time constants and a similar relation to cycloversion. The existence of DVD was also demonstrated in normal subjects, supporting the hypothesis that DVD reflects a natural tendency of the eyes and is restrained by normal binocular vision.

Guyton et al. also used scleral search coil eye movement recordings to investigate DVD. Analysis of the simultaneous vertical and torsional eye movements in their recordings showed that the vertical versions in their patients were largely mediated by the oblique muscles in the fixating eye and by the vertical rectus muscles in the nonfixating eye. Vertical vergence movements were largely mediated by the oblique muscles in both eyes. Since latent nystagmus is strongly associated with DVD, Guyton et al. theorized that DVD might serve to damp latent nystagmus or stabilize the fixating eye when latent nystagmus was present. They found that the slow phase of latent nystagmus is always conjugate for the two eyes, with the fixating eye usually drifting in, down, and intorting and the nonfixating eye drifting out, down, and extorting. These eye muscle recordings indicated that latent nystagmus has both a horizontal and a cyclovertical component. Convergence is often used to damp the horizontal component. The cyclovertical eye movements in DVD appear to damp the cyclovertical component of the latent nystagmus. The damping occurs by way of a vertical vergence involving activation of the superior oblique muscle in the fixating eye that tends to cause depression, intorsion, and abduction. In the nonfixating eye, the inferior oblique muscle causes elevation, extorsion, and abduction.

Simultaneously, vertical and horizontal versions occur to neutralize the tendency toward abduction and depression of the fixating eye in order to maintain fixation. The upward version is produced by the inferior oblique muscle of the fixating eye and by the superior rectus muscle of the nonfixating eye, elevating the nonfixating eye still further. The horizontal version occurs toward the nonfixating eye, causing the nonfixating eye to abduct still farther. The end result is that the fixating eye continues to fixate, although slightly intorted, and the nonfixating eye is elevated, extorted, and abducted. Convergence compensation for the horizontal component of the latent nystagmus, if present, can negate the abduction of the nonfixating eye. This fact may explain why DHD is seen less prominently than DVD in most patients.

Brodsky has further refined the phylogenetic theories about the origin of DSC. He reminds us that in the course of evolution, primitive responses to external stimuli are suppressed by newer neurologic reflexes. When these newer systems fail to function properly, primitive reflexes may reappear. Brodsky theorizes that DVD is a dorsal light reflex in which asymmetric visual input to the two eyes evokes a vertical divergence movement of the eyes. This primitive visuovestibular reflex functions as a righting response to restore vertical orientation in lateral-eyed lower animals by equalizing binocular vision input. The dorsal light reflex is suppressed in humans, but can manifest as DVD when early-onset strabismus precludes normal binocular development. Van Rijn has pointed out that Brodsky's theory does not offer an explanation for isolated DTD and DHD.

One additional causation theory for DSC deserves mention. In 1985, Lang theorized that the organization of the oculomotor nucleus may help explain DVD; he restated this hypothesis in 1995. At the time of Bielschowsky, the *Bernheimer scheme* was accepted for the organization of the oculomotor nucleus, in which the nerves that innervated the eye muscles were uncrossed. It was not until 1953 that Warwick showed that the paired oculomotor nucleus has crossed motor neurons for the superior rectus muscle and uncrossed motor neurons for the medial and inferior rectus muscles and inferior oblique muscle. Bielschowsky had recognized that the slow elevation movements of DVD can be elicited by a difference in the incidence of light in the two eyes, as shown with the darkening glass wedge in front of the fixating eye. Light fibers subserving the pupillary mechanism do not reach the lateral geniculate nucleus, but go by the posterior commissure immediately to the pretectum and from there to the nucleus of the third nerve.

Lang further theorized that since it is known that in the vestibular centers for oculomotor movement there may be an unequal tonus, what is true for vestibular centers may also be true for the oculomotor nucleus. When one part of the oculomotor nucleus, because of light imbalance, has a higher tonus than the other, a slow sursumduction of the contralateral eye and an infraduction of the ipsilateral eye are induced. Since binocularity is interrupted, this movement is not controlled by the visual cortex or the brain stem centers for vision.

It is evident from the complicated etiologic discussion above that DSC remains an enigma.

COMMENT

Marshall M. Parks, MD

I doubt that DSC serves any useful function, and probably represents the residue resulting from an absence of macular binocular vision and a poor hold on extramacular binocular vision. Visual attention may be able to offer some control over the deviation among those who enjoy either normal or abnormal retinal correspondence (NRC or ARC) extramacular fusion; but in the absence of visual attention, the worse of these disorders is apparent.

In DSC patients devoid of the extramacular binocular vision reflex, the dissociated deviations are constantly present, regardless of the state of visual attention. I have had the experience of testing DSC patients while they wore Bagolini glasses. Some are very clever in switching fixation voluntarily from eye to eye and in voluntarily maintaining extramacular fusion one moment and surrendering it the next moment, revealing a large DVD. While fusing, they simultaneously see the streak on both retinas by describing an X; but the next moment, voluntarily surrendering their fusion, the streak is seen only by the fixating eye, and the streak on the updrifting eye disappears. Upon switching fixation, the reverse happens. As the patient re-fuses, the vertical tropia disappears and the X reappears. On questioning, the patient can locate the break in the streak, projecting onto the nonfixating eye's macula, which can be transferred from eye to eye by switching the fixation, all the while continuously viewing the X with both eyes remaining on the level. Such bright patients can achieve a remarkable level of voluntary control of the various reflexes necessary to produce these findings. To them, it becomes an entertaining parlor trick.

This convinces me that the dissociated deviations are purposeless movements of the eyes resulting from absence of macular binocular vision and from either lack of development or intermittent suspension of the extramacular binocular vision reflex. Surgery never cures DSC; it simply reduces the conspicuousness of the deviation associated with visual inattention or absence of extramacular binocular vision.

INCIDENCE OF THE COMPLEX

DSC is present in 60% to 80% of all congenital esotropia patients but can also be seen in association with other forms of strabismus. If searched for diligently, DVD (the most commonly recognized component of DSC) probably represents the most common hyperdeviation seen in a strabismus practice. Helveston found DVD in 11.1% of 1000 consecutive patients with strabismus or nystagmus. Among esotropia patients, the incidence was 14%. Dissociated vertical deviation was found in 8.7% of patients with exotropia and 7.2% of patients with hypertropia.

Dissociated horizontal deviation is much less commonly seen than DVD. However, one report documented DHD prominent enough to require surgery in 5% of patients with a history of congenital esotropia. The incidence figures for DHD are increasing since it is now being recognized more easily and distinguished more accurately from intermittent exotropia.

The incidence of each of the three components of DSC (DVD, DHD, DTD) is determined in part by how carefully the examiner searches for them. The same holds true for latent nystagmus, which nearly always accompanies DSC regardless of whether the DSC is severe or subtle.

OCULAR MANIFESTATIONS OF THE COMPLEX

Dissociated strabismus complex is almost always a bilateral but asymmetric condition (Fig. 4–2). In an analysis of 170 patients, von Noorden found bilaterality in 86% and asymmetry in 91%. When a unilateral dissociated deviation is detected initially, careful observation over several examinations usually reveals an asymmetric bilateral DSC rather than a truly unilateral finding. Dissociated strabismus complex may manifest spontaneously or may be controlled by binocular fusion mechanisms and remain latent. Even though it may be manifest often, DSC nearly always remains intermittent and varies with the state of attention of the individual. Visual inattention or, perhaps more accurately, active fixation by one eye in the complete absence of any attempt at binocular function often produces a larger deviation than can be measured by even prolonged alternate cover testing, and variability is the rule. Deviations can appear small and well controlled on one visit, only to be large and to manifest spontaneously a short time later.

Suppression of the deviated eye prevents diplopia. At times, however, red-lens testing can elicit diplopia. For DVD, the red light appears below the white light regardless of which eye it is placed before. As stated above, dissociated horizontal and torsional movements are now recognized with greater frequency. A DVD,

A 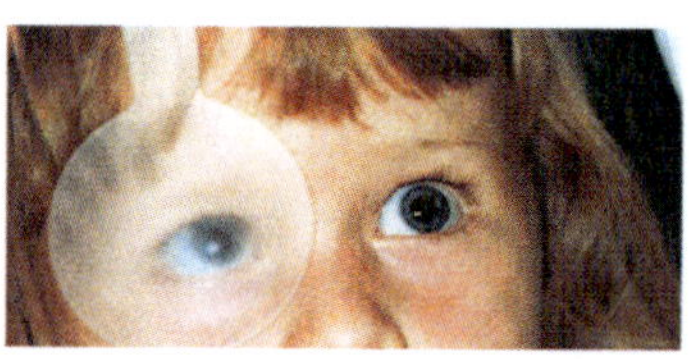 B 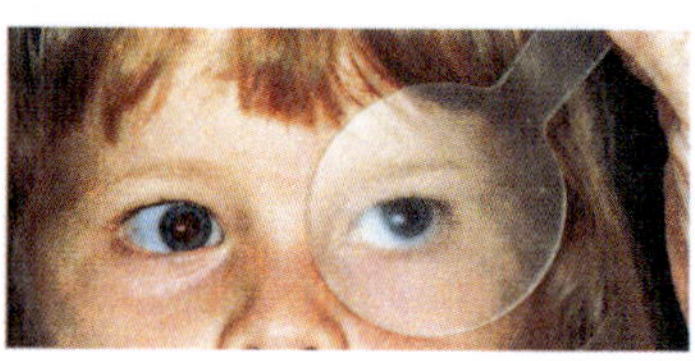

Figure 4–2. Bilateral asymmetric dissociated strabismus complex. Cover testing showed (*A*) moderate dissociated vertical deviation (DVD) and dissociated torsional deviation (DTD) in the right eye and (*B*) marked DVD with moderate dissociated horizontal deviation (DHD) and DTD in the left eye. Latent nystagmus was seen with cover testing of either eye.

however, remains the predominant manifestation in most cases of DSC. For that reason, the recognition of DVD is given more emphasis in this chapter.

True vertical tropias can be quantitated by placing base-down prisms before the higher eye or base-up prisms before the lower eye until all refixation movements are neutralized. The alternate cover test reveals these refixation movements to be upward in one eye and downward in the other eye, in accordance with Hering's law of equal motor innervation. The hyperdeviation of DVD is not a true vertical tropia since no corresponding hypotropia is present in the fellow eye. Hering's law, therefore, does not appear to apply to DVD (although Guyton has made the argument that each of the various components of the DSC response does indeed obey Hering's law). The absence of upward refixation movements in either eye on alternate cover testing best distinguishes DVD from true vertical tropia. In addition, the upward drift of DVD is very slow (2° to 20° per second) compared to movements seen with true hypertropia (200° to 400° per second).

In addition, DVD is more complex, usually having associated DHD, DTD, and latent nystagmus movements. When attempting to quantify DVD, the examiner must measure each eye separately. Prisms are placed base-down before the eye to be measured until it no longer rises behind the cover. The measurement end point is not a true neutralization, since the fellow eye will have been rendered hypotropic by the prisms. Even with this method, DVD measurements are variable from day to day, and even from moment to moment, and tend to increase with prolonged occlusion. For these reasons, a subjective 1+ to 4+ scale is often used to describe DVD. Close observation usually reveals extorsion and abduction as the eye with DVD rises and intorsion and adduction on recovery toward primary position. Latent nystagmus is also present in the majority of these patients.

Dissociated strabismus complex marked almost exclusively by DHD, with very little DVD, can occur (Fig. 4–3). Attempting to neutralize DHD with prisms poses the same problems just discussed with DVD, except that the prisms are placed horizontally. Dissociated horizontal deviation is distinguished from intermittent exotropia by the speed of the abducting movement, associated DTD, and the absence of true neutralization with prisms. In addition, a rapid alternate cover test often reveals a microesotropia, but a slow alternate cover test (allowing the eye with DHD to completely dissociate) reveals the exodeviated posture behind the cover.

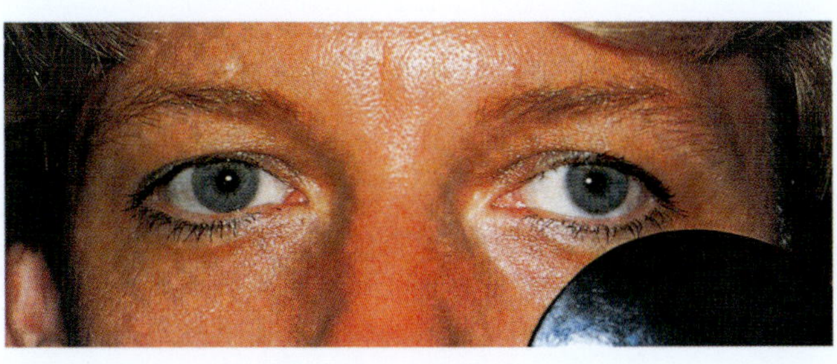

Figure 4–3. Dissociated strabismus complex manifesting almost exclusively as dissociated horizontal deviation (DHD). As the cover was removed from the left eye, left DHD and dissociated torsional deviation (DTD) could be seen. Only DTD movement was seen when the cover was placed over the right eye. Latent nystagmus was present when either eye was covered.

Normally, DSC is not seen in association with high-grade stereopsis and macular binocular vision. If any binocular cooperation is detected, it is usually peripheral binocularity, as in the monofixation syndrome of Parks. Although DSC is usually seen in association with previously treated horizontal strabismus, it can also be seen in patients with poor stereopsis but no history of previous surgery. These patients often have primary monofixation syndrome and sometimes are found to be first-degree relatives of patients with congenital esotropia.

Dissociated strabismus complex can coexist with oblique muscle dysfunction. Dissociated vertical deviation and inferior oblique overaction (IOOA) are both very common in congenital esotropia patients. Dissociated vertical deviation can simulate IOOA when, in lateral gaze, the nose acts as an occluder, allowing a latent DVD to become manifest. If a true hypertropia is present in lateral gaze, IOOA is present. If DVD is evident in primary gaze but much less elevation is present behind the cover when the eye is in abduction, contralateral IOOA is suspected. If elevation is much less when the eye is in adduction, ipsilateral superior oblique overaction (SOOA) is suspected. In other words, incomitant DVD implies the presence of oblique muscle dysfunction. To verify the coexistence of DVD and IOOA, the DVD is allowed to become fully manifest behind the cover. Without removing the cover, the examiner looks for elevation as the eye moves into adduction. In addition, a lowering of the eye is seen in abduction if the IOOA is bilateral.

The Bielschowsky phenomenon is unique to DSC. It can be demonstrated in more than 50% of patients with a prominent DVD, especially if it is asymmetric and amblyopia is present. Downward movement of the elevated, occluded eye occurs when filters of increasing density are placed before the fixating eye. The eye behind the cover may even come to rest below primary position. A Bagolini graded red filter bar is useful to elicit the Bielschowsky phenomenon. Alternatively, two polarized filters used with many near stereopsis tests can be rotated on one another before the fixating eye to create a darkening filter. The phenomenon can also be demonstrated in the horizontal plane in patients with a prominent DHD.

A prominent head tilt can be seen in association with DSC. The deviation should be measured first in the preferred head posture and then with forced head tilt in the opposite direction. If DVD or DHD is increased or becomes manifest with the forced head-tilt maneuver, it is likely contributing to the anomalous posture. When this occurs, the head posture is improved by surgical procedures that help to reduce the DSC. While DVD is usually worsened by head tilt to the contralateral side (the opposite of that found in superior oblique muscle palsy), the converse can sometimes be true.

TREATMENT FOR DISSOCIATED VERTICAL DEVIATION

Dissociated vertical deviation rarely causes diplopia, but it can be disfiguring since even small hyperdeviations will appear prominent as sclera begins to be visible at the lower eyelid margin. Symptomatic DVD is usually treated surgically. Occasionally, when DVD is unilateral, the fixating eye can be blurred optically to promote a switch in fixation, thus preventing the dissociated drift of that eye.

COMMENT
Michael X. Repka, MD

I agree with Dr. Wilson that DVD rarely causes diplopia, but in some patients it is associated with an uncomfortable feeling when the eyes are deviated. This too can be a reason for proceeding with corrective surgery in addition to the hyperdeviation.

Some surgeons prefer to treat DVD with inferior rectus muscle resections, but most prefer to recess the superior rectus muscles. Unilateral surgery may be indicated if DVD manifests spontaneously in only one eye, especially when a difference of two or more lines in visual acuity is present between the eyes. Unilateral superior rectus muscle recessions for these patients typically range from 5.0 to 9.0 mm and usually result in an ipsilateral hypotropia that lasts for days to weeks. Fewer undercorrections occur when unilateral surgery is performed for DVD. However, a switch in fixation may occur, resulting in manifest DVD in the previously asymptomatic eye. Therefore, bilateral surgery is advocated by some surgeons for all DVD patients either symmetrically or asymmetrically, with the amount of surgery on each eye being determined by the severity of the DVD in that eye. When performing bilateral superior rectus muscle recession for DVD, this author prefers large, symmetric recessions (7.0 to 10.0 mm), regardless of the asymmetry of the DVD severity.

COMMENT
David A. Plager, MD

It is worth emphasizing that unilateral surgery for DVD, even when marked DVD asymmetry is present, often leads to an unmasking of the DVD in the opposite eye. Unless there is very poor vision in one eye that will preclude it from ever taking up fixation, I prefer to do a preemptive strike in the preferred eye. For instance, the worse eye would get a large superior rectus recession of perhaps 9.0 mm and the fellow eye a smaller (4.0 to 7.0 mm) recession, depending on the degree of asymmetry in the DVD.

Posterior fixation sutures (fadenoperation) placed 12.0 to 15.0 mm posterior to the superior rectus insertion, either alone or in combination with superior rectus muscle recession, have been advocated as an effective treatment for DVD. (For a discussion of the fadenoperation, see Chapter 5, "Paralytic Strabismus.") However, Esswein et al. reported that although the effectiveness of 3.0 to 5.0 mm superior rectus muscle recession combined with a posterior fixation suture was excellent at 6 months postoperatively (87% corrected or improved), a failure rate of 55% was documented 3 years after surgery. In contrast, the success rate of 7.0

to 9.0 mm superior rectus muscle recession diminished only slightly over time, with 86% corrected or improved at 6 months, 80% at 1 year, 77% at 2 years, and 72% at 3 years. Most surgeons have abandoned posterior fixation sutures of the superior rectus as a treatment for DVD.

Anterior transposition of the inferior oblique muscle, a modified recession procedure developed to treat marked IOOA, has also been shown to reduce DVD. (For details of anterior transposition, see Chapter 3, "Oblique Muscle Dysfunction.") This procedure is recommended as a treatment for marked bilateral IOOA, especially when mild DVD is also present or DVD is likely to manifest in the future. Inferior oblique muscle anterior transposition alone may be inadequate for DVD of 15 prism diopters (Δ) or more in severity. Although some surgeons have reported resection of the inferior oblique combined with anterior transposition, care must be taken to avoid marked up-gaze deficiency or a T pattern, which can result when the inferior oblique muscle is transposed too far anteriorly or spread out too far laterally.

Mims and Wood used interior oblique anterior transposition as a prophylactic procedure for DVD in 61 children with congenital esotropia and bilateral IOOA. With an average follow-up of 27 months, only one patient needed surgery for DVD compared to nine in a control group of congenital esotropia patients who had not undergone inferior oblique muscle surgery.

The following scheme is recommended for DVD surgery:

1. *For DVD alone:* large superior rectus muscle recessions (7.0 to 10.0 mm) done symmetrically and bilaterally even if the DVD is asymmetric
2. *For mild to moderate DVD (less than 15Δ) associated with IOOA:* symmetric bilateral inferior oblique muscle anterior transposition even with, or 2.0 mm anterior to, the lateral border of the inferior rectus insertion
3. *For moderate to severe DVD (greater than 15Δ) associated with IOOA:* combined 7.0 to 8.0 mm bilateral superior rectus muscle recession and bilateral symmetric inferior oblique muscle anterior transposition up to, but not beyond, the insertion of the inferior rectus muscle

COMMENT

Michael X. Repka, MD

For mild to moderate DVD with IOOA, I use anteriorization with the nasal aspect of the inferior oblique sewn to sclera level with and 2.0 mm temporal to the inferior rectus insertion. The lateral edge of the inferior oblique muscle is recessed an additional 1.0 to 2.0 mm so that those posterior fibers are not excessively anteriorized. For severe DVD, I do not weaken both of the elevators at the same operation. I have been uncomfortable with the severe up-gaze limitation and the remarkable amount of lid retraction that often ensue.

COMMENT

Edward G. Buckley, MD

The amount of superior rectus recession depends on whether or not inferior oblique surgery has also been performed. Large superior rectus recessions after bilateral inferior oblique surgery can result in a significant elevation deficit. While this is not a problem functionally, it can cause bilateral lid retraction, which can be cosmetically unacceptable. I prefer to keep bilateral superior rectus recessions to 6.0 mm or less in situations where bilateral inferior oblique surgery has been performed.

In performing superior rectus recessions for DVD, I favor the hangback technique. This avoids the problem of suturing through the superior oblique tendon or, in large superior rectus recessions, redirecting the superior oblique tendon posteriorly.

In patients with DVD and overacting inferior obliques, an alternative surgical approach to anteriorization is simple myectomy of the inferior oblique muscle combined with bilateral superior rectus recessions. This *bilateral elevator weakness* procedure is extremely effective in eliminating both the IOOA and the DVD. It eliminates the risk of antielevation syndrome, which can occur after inferior oblique anteriorization surgery. It is also less likely to give an asymmetric result.

In patients with asymmetric DVD and no fixation preference after bilateral superior rectus recessions, I prefer to perform a fadenoperation on the offending superior rectus. The fadenoperation needs to be at least 20.0 mm posterior to the limbus and preferably farther. This requires placing the suture through the superior oblique tendon to avoid superior oblique dysfunction caused by redirecting the tendon.

COMMENT

David A. Plager, MD

While the hangback technique is technically easier than a conventional large superior rectus recession, one wonders whether the muscle really hangs back as far as we intend. It appears to be well back on the operating table, with the eye held in infraduction; but when the patient awakens and elevates the eye to a normal position, the attachments to the superior oblique on the underside and the levator complex on its superior surface may pull the superior rectus farther anteriorly, therefore diminishing the intended effect.

Resection of the inferior rectus muscle should not be overlooked as an option. Surgeons, including myself, are somewhat reluctant to use this option, probably because of concerns about elevating the lower lid position with a large resection; but in the few patients on whom I have performed this procedure, the results have been encouraging. Particular care must be taken to aggressively dissect the inferior rectus from surrounding intermuscular septum, attachments to the inferior oblique, and lower lid retractors while avoiding the vortex veins on either side and not violating the fat pad to avoid associated complications.

TREATMENT FOR DISSOCIATED HORIZONTAL DEVIATION

In 1991, Wilson and McClatchey recommended lateral rectus muscle recession for the treatment of manifest DHD and reported good results in six patients with 5 to 27 months of postoperative follow-up. A unilateral recession was used in five of the six patients, because manifest DHD was seen in only one eye. This is in contrast to DVD, which usually requires bilateral surgery. In 2000, Wilson et al. reported 33 consecutive patients who underwent surgery to correct DHD. Of these patients, 25 (78%) underwent a single operation, 7 (22%) underwent two operations, and 2 of those 7 (6% of the total) underwent three operations to control DHD or horizontal strabismus accompanying the DHD. Most of the patients (75%) had a history of congenital esotropia. Only 4 (15%) of the 27 patients initially operated on unilaterally for DHD required DHD surgery in the fellow eye. (In contrast, all three of the patients in this DHD treatment group who underwent unilateral DVD surgery eventually needed an operation on the fellow eye for DVD.) Bilateral surgery for DHD appeared to be necessary only in patients with combined exotropia at distance and DHD or large bilateral DHD with alternating fixation.

The following surgical approach to a DHD is recommended:

1. *For unilateral DHD measured or estimated at greater than 15Δ:* an ipsilateral lateral rectus muscle recession of 7.0 mm. The recession is reduced to 5.0 mm if the DHD measures 15Δ or less. The lateral rectus muscle recession is reduced if the lateral rectus muscle has been previously resected. This last reduction is based on forced ductions performed at the time of the DHD surgery. More reduction is indicated when the previously resected lateral rectus muscle is tight.
2. *For esotropia greater than 10Δ coexisting with DHD:* the lateral rectus muscle recession is reduced to 5.0 mm or the esotropia is treated concomitantly with the DHD. This may entail bilateral medial rectus muscle recession along with unilateral lateral rectus muscle recession or bilateral medial rectus muscle posterior fixation sutures along with unilateral lateral rectus muscle recession.
3. *For exotropia at distance and coexisting DHD or when DHD is frequently manifest in either eye as a result of alternate fixation:* bilateral lateral rectus muscle recession is recommended.

ACKNOWLEDGMENT

This chapter has been expanded with permission from Wilson ME, Serafino, M: Dissociated strabismus complex. *Contemporary Ophthalmol* 2002; 1:1–5.

Suggested Readings

Bielschowsky A: *Lectures on Motor Anomalies.* Hanover, NH: Dartmouth Publications; 1956, 34.

Braverman DE, Scott WE: Surgical correction of dissociated vertical deviations. *J Pediatr Ophthalmol Strabismus* 1977; 14:337–342.

Brodsky MC: Dissociated vertical divergence: a righting reflex gone wrong. *Arch Ophthalmol* 1999; 117:1216–1222.

Brown HW: Dissociated vertical anomalies. In: Arruga A, ed: *International Strabismus Symposium: an evaluation of the present status of orthoptics, pleoptics and related diagnostic and treatment regimes.* New York: S Karger; 1968, 175–179.

Calhoun JH: Dissociated vertical deviation. In: Spaeth GL, Catz LJ, eds: *Current Therapy in Ophthalmic Surgery.* Toronto and Philadelphia: BC Decker; 1989, 286–287.

Cheeseman EW Jr, Guyton DL: Vertical fusional vergence: the key to dissociated vertical deviation. *Arch Ophthalmol* 1999; 117:1188–1191.

Enke ES, Stewart SA, Scott WE, et al: The prevalence of dissociated horizontal deviations in congenital esotropia. *Am Orthopt J* 1994; 44:109–111.

Enright JT: Unexpected role of the oblique muscles in human vertical fusional reflex. *J Physiol* 1992; 451:279–293.

Esswein MB, von Noorden GK, Coburn A: Comparison of surgical methods in the treatment of dissociated vertical deviation. *Am J Ophthalmol* 1992; 113:287–290.

Guyton DL: Dissociated vertical deviation: etiology, mechanism, and associated phenomena. *J Am Assoc Pediatr Ophthalmol Strabismus* 2000; 4:131–144.

Guyton DL, Cheeseman EW Jr, Ellis FJ, et al: Dissociated vertical deviation: an exaggerated normal eye movement used to damp cyclovertical latent nystagmus. *Trans Am Ophthalmol Soc* 1998; 96:389–424; discussion 424–429.

Helveston EM: A-exotropia, alternating sursumduction, and superior oblique overaction. *Am J Ophthalmol* 1969; 67:377–380.

Helveston EM: Dissociated vertical deviation: a clinical and laboratory study. *Trans Am Ophthalmol Soc* 1980; 78:734–779.

Lang J: The congenital strabismus syndrome. *Proceedings of the International Symposium on Strabismus and Amblyopia.* April 14–18, 1985, Tel Aviv, Israel. Paris: CERES; 1985: 1–7.

Lang J: *Strabismus*, 4th ed. Bern: Huber; 1995.

Magoon E, Cruciger M, Jampolsky A: Dissociated vertical deviation: an asymmetric condition treated with large bilateral superior rectus recession. *J Pediatr Ophthalmol Strabismus* 1982; 19:152–156.

Mims JL III, Wood RC: Bilateral anterior transportation of the inferior obliques. *Arch Ophthalmol* 1989; 107:41–44.

Raab EL: Dissociative vertical deviation. *J Pediatr Ophthalmol Strabismus* 1970; 7:146–151.

Rosenbaum AL, Santiago AP, eds: *Clinical Strabismus Management: Principles and Surgical Techniques.* Philadelphia: WB Saunders Co; 1999, 237–248.

Scobee RG: *The Oculorotary Muscles.* St Louis: CV Mosby Co; 1947, 142–154.

Stegall FW: Dissociated vertical deviations: current research. *Am Orthopt J* 1981; 31: 40–46.

van Rijn LJ: The cause of dissociated vertical deviation. *Strabismus* 2000; 8:53–54.

van Rijn LJ, Collewijn H: Eye torsion associated with disparity-induced vertical vergence in humans. *Vis Res* 1994; 34:2307–2316.

van Rijn LJ, Simonsz HJ, ten Tusscher MP: Dissociated vertical deviation and eye torsion: relation to disparity-induced vertical vergence. *Strabismus* 1997; 5:13–20.

van Rijn LJ, ten Tusscher MP, de Jong I, et al: Asymmetrical vertical phorias indicating dissociated vertical deviation in subjects with normal binocular vision. *Vis Res* 1998; 38:2973–2978.

Varn MM, Saunders RA, Wilson ME: Combined bilateral superior rectus muscle recession and inferior oblique muscle weakening for dissociated vertical deviation. *J Am Assoc Pediatr Ophthalmol Strabismus* 1997; 1:134–137.

Verhoeff FH: Occlusion hypertropia. *Arch Ophthalmol* 1941; 25:780–795.

von Noorden GK: *Binocular Vision and Ocular Motility: Theory and Management of Strabismus*, 5th ed. St Louis: CV Mosby Co; 1996: 361–367.

Warwick R: Oculomotor organization. In: Bender M, ed: *The Oculomotor System.* New York: Harper & Row; 1964, 173–201.

Wilson ME: The dissociated strabismus complex. *Binocul Vis* 1993; 8:45–46.

Wilson ME: Dissociated strabismus. In: Tasman W, Jaeger EA, eds: *Duane's Clinical Ophthalmology*, Vol 1. Philadelphia: JB Lippincott Co; 1998, chap 18.

Wilson ME, Hutchinson AK, Saunders RA: Outcomes from surgical treatment for dissociated horizontal deviation. *J Am Assoc Pediatr Ophthalmol Strabismus* 2000; 4:94–101.

Wilson ME, McClatchey SK: Dissociated horizontal deviation. *J Pediatr Ophthalmol Strabismus* 1991; 28:90–95.

Wilson ME, Parks MM: Primary inferior oblique overaction in congenital esotropia, accommodative esotropia, and intermittent exotropia. *Ophthalmology* 1989; 96:950–955; discussion 956–957.

5

Paralytic Strabismus

EDWARD G. BUCKLEY

The treatment of ocular motility disorders, which occur after injury to one or more of the motor nerves to the extraocular muscles, presents a therapeutic challenge. The goal of treatment is to create a large area of single binocular vision that is centered around the primary-gaze position while preserving as much single vision in the reading position as possible. In most cases of paralytic strabismus, a variety of surgical approaches can be used. However, to achieve high patient satisfaction, the successful procedure must result in an area of single binocular vision that is large enough to permit normal gaze function. Careful analysis of the ocular motility deficit, with special emphasis on the amount and direction of extraocular muscle dysfunction, is crucial in selecting the appropriate surgical procedure.

Paralytic strabismus is difficult to treat because the amount of misalignment varies, depending on the direction of gaze. For example, a patient with a right sixth nerve palsy has a large esotropia on right gaze, a smaller esotropia in the primary position, and often no esotropia on left gaze. The incomitance of the motility abnormality makes it impossible to correct with prisms or standard strabismus techniques, which work best when the amount of misalignment is equal in all gaze positions.

In the above example, a standard recession and resection procedure can eliminate the esotropia in the primary position, but a residual esotropia will remain on right gaze and a new exotropia will be created on left gaze. Postoperatively, the patient's diplopia changes from crossed on left gaze to uncrossed on right gaze. This variable deviation makes it difficult for the patient to maintain single binocular vision. Minimizing this type of result will increase both patient function and patient satisfaction.

A second complicating factor in treating paralytic strabismus is the possibility that horizontal, vertical, and torsional components to the deviation may be present. This is especially true in third nerve palsies, where horizontal and vertical muscles are often simultaneously affected, and in fourth nerve palsies, where torsional issues occur. In such circumstances, all aspects of the motility disturbance must be addressed to get a satisfactory result.

Finally, in patients with long-standing paralysis, the ocular motility defect may have a restrictive component due to contracture of the antagonist muscle. The greater the paralysis, the more likely the opposing muscle will tighten over time. Recognition of this phenomenon is important because any planned surgical procedure must deal with the induced restriction.

SURGICAL PRINCIPLES

Since the major problem in paralytic strabismus is incomitance, the best surgical procedure will be one that has an incomitant result. That is, the corrective effect of the operation will be greater in one field of gaze than in another. The appropriate incomitant strabismus surgery can be developed by taking two fundamental principles into consideration:

1. The first principle is to *improve the ocular rotation* in the involved eye. This can usually be achieved by increasing the action of the involved muscle through a resection or tuck-type procedure, creating an alternate force vector (often necessary in complete paralysis) by an extraocular muscle transposition procedure or by weakening the antagonist muscle's function.
2. The second principle is to *create a matching defect* in the sound eye. This is usually necessary because it is impossible to restore normal function to the paralytic muscle. Since diplopia results from an imbalance in the coordinated effort between the eyes, the normal eye rotation must be matched to whatever function can be achieved in the paretic eye. This usually is accomplished by weakening the yoke muscle of the paretic muscle in the uninvolved eye.

Factors in Surgical Planning. With the above principles in mind, the two most important factors in evaluating a patient with paralytic strabismus are the *amount of residual function* of the paralytic muscle and the *direction of gaze in which the deviation is greatest*. By assessment of these two fundamental parameters, a surgical schema to treat patients with paralytic strabismus can be created (Fig. 5–1).

Residual muscle function can be graded on a three-part scale:

1. *Mild* function is indicative of minimal limitation and only slightly decreased movement in the field of greatest action of the muscle. Mild residual muscle functions can be associated with fairly large deviations, so it is not the size of the deviation but rather the function of the muscle that is important to assess.
2. *Moderate* decrease in residual muscle function usually indicates a functionally significant limitation. Muscle function may be reduced as much as 50% to 75%, but it is definitely still present.

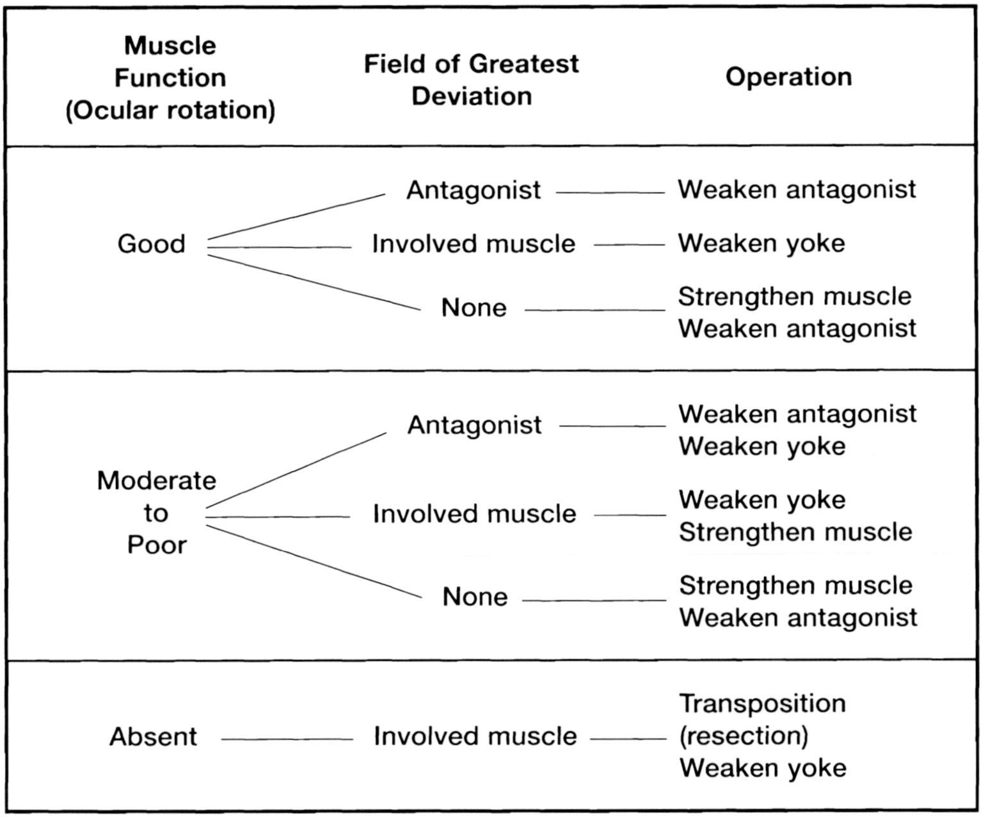

Figure 5–1. Surgical strategy chart to treat paralytic strabismus. The most important clinical assessment factors are residual function of the paralytic muscle and gaze direction in which the eyes are most out of alignment. Combining these two factors results in a suggested surgical approach that maximizes and centers the area of single binocular vision.

3. *Severe* limitation indicates no function of the muscle at all. The eye cannot be moved into the normal field of action of the muscle. An example is no abduction of the eye past midline in a patient with a sixth nerve palsy.

COMMENT

Michael X. Repka, MD

For a patient with paralytic strabismus, I measure the limitation of ductions on an arc perimeter at each visit. I use this measurement as an indicator of improvement, deterioration, or stabilization longitudinally. The measurement is also helpful in planning a surgical procedure. Alternatively, the force generation test is helpful in deciding between a large recess-resect operation and a transposition surgery. The test is performed by placing forceps on the globe and asking the patient to look into the field of limitation. The examiner feels the globe through the forceps for any muscular function as the patient looks into the field of the paretic muscle. The presence of some force generation prompts me to choose the recess-resect operation rather than a transposition.

The *field of greatest deviation* is also characterized in one of three ways and can usually be easily identified: The greatest deviation is (*1*) in the direction of the involved muscle, (*2*) in the direction of the antagonist muscle, or (*3*) equal in both directions. The last usually implies contracture of the antagonist muscle and is the easiest to treat.

These two variables, muscle function and field of greatest deviation, while being assessed as independent, actually are not. It would be very difficult to have a severe limitation of muscle function and no field of greatest deviation. By the application of these two parameters, an operation is designed to improve or eliminate the incomitance. The other important factor in the operation's design *is to minimize the creation of a misalignment in a gaze position where preoperatively it did not exist.*

The goal is to preserve all areas of single binocular vision that were present preoperatively while at the same time eliminating areas of diplopia. Because this is often not possible, a secondary goal is to minimize the number of new diplopic areas created by the surgical procedure. This is an extremely important point. Patients are most distressed when previous areas of single binocular vision have been eliminated in the attempt to improve the diplopia in other fields of gaze. This becomes especially disconcerting if the resultant field of single binocular vision is very narrow or if the diplopia changes direction with small gaze changes (that is, esotropia in one field and exotropia in another).

The schema outlined in Figure 5–1 is based on an assessment of these two factors. This is the foundation for the surgical treatment of the specific types of paralytic strabismus to be discussed.

SURGICAL CONSIDERATIONS

Fadenoperation. The fadenoperation, also known as *posterior fixation suture*, is ideally suited to treating paralytic strabismus. The primary benefit of the fadenoperation is selective limitation of ocular rotation. This makes it most useful in correcting incomitant strabismus, especially if primary-position alignment is satisfactory and change is required in only one direction of gaze (Fig. 5–2). Since this is often the case in treating paralytic strabismus, this operation can be used in place of recession or in combination with recession to achieve the maximum effect.

The fadenoperation can also be used to eliminate or prevent iatrogenic incomitant vertical strabismus after maximum muscle recession. This may occur in patients who have had an inferior rectus recession for a double elevator palsy and are now orthophoric in the primary position but have an iatrogenic vertical deviation on down gaze due to the recessed inferior rectus. A fadenoperation on the contralateral inferior rectus can often improve or eliminate the down-gaze diplopia.

COMMENT

Gunter K. von Noorden, MD

The German *fadenoperation* is imprecise and misleading: *imprecise*, because it translates literally as a surgical procedure in which a *faden*—that is, a surgical suture, thread, or stitch—is used (sutures are used in most surgical

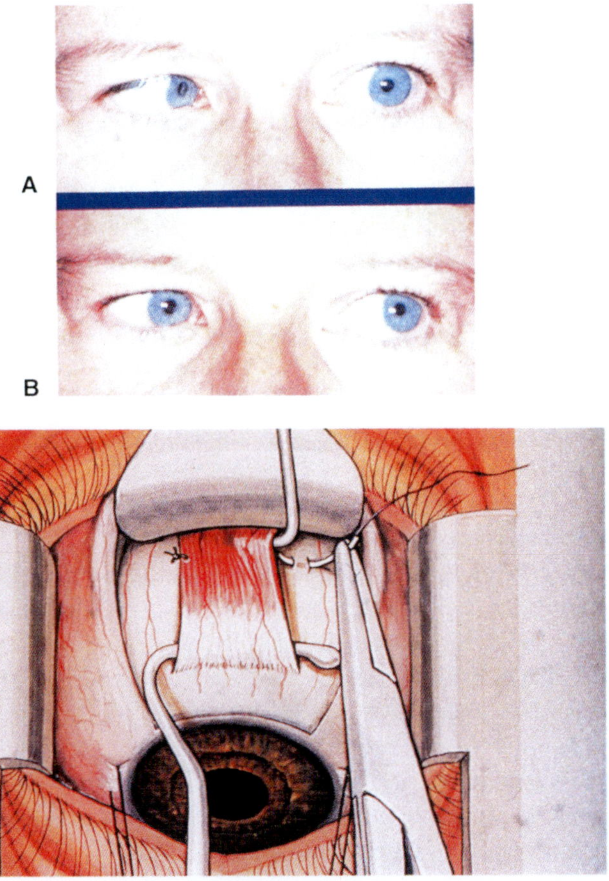

Figure 5–2. Fadenoperation for left sixth nerve palsy. (*A*) A patient had undergone a transposition procedure, with relocation of the inferior and superior rectus muscles to the lateral rectus on the left. Postoperatively, the patient still has esodeviation on left gaze. (*B*) Patient after fadenoperation on the medial rectus of the right eye. Limitation has been created on the right eye, which allows a wider area of single binocular vision before diplopia occurs on left gaze. (*C*) A fadenoperation is performed by suturing the rectus muscle to the eye 12.0 mm posterior to the insertion with nonabsorbable suture. The result is to create an effective new insertion at the suture location without otherwise weakening the muscle, which results in decreased rotation in the muscle's field of action.

procedures); *misleading* because this same term was introduced by Dieffenbach in 1842 for an entirely different procedure, namely passage of a traction suture through the insertion of the lateral rectus muscle and fixation to the opposite side of the face, after advancing the previously myotomized medial rectus muscle in patients with a consecutive exotropia. It is unfortunate and has caused confusion that Cüppers reintroduced the same term for his operation, and I see no reason for using it in the English language, especially since more descriptive and correct terms, such as *retroequatorial myopexy* and *posterior fixation suture*, are available.

Transposition Procedures. Transpositions provide a movement force in the direction of the transposed muscles that is not active but passive, much like a spring. This passive force can be modulated by the antagonist muscle to allow controlled movement of the eye. The saccadic velocity in the direction of transposed muscles is significantly decreased from normal, and patients still experience difficulties when looking in the direction of the transposed muscles, especially if a fast movement is required. Regardless, transpositions are usually superior to resections when muscle function is totally absent, provided that the transposed muscles are functioning normally. There are a variety of transposition procedures to choose from, including the full-tendon, Knapp, and Hummelsheim, but the full tendon is preferred (Fig. 5–3).

Several modifications to the full-tendon transposition procedure have been shown to increase its effectiveness. Buckley uses a nonabsorbable suture to attach the edges of the transposed muscle to the paralytic muscle (Fig. 5–4). Foster described a similar technique in which the suture is placed approximately 8.0 mm posterior to the new insertion, along the border of the transposed muscle closest to the paralyzed muscle. The edge of the transposed muscle is sutured to the globe at this location. This redirects more of the transposed muscle's force vector in the direction of the paralytic muscle (Fig. 5–5).

In the Knapp procedure, the entire rectus muscle is transposed to the paralytic muscle. Unlike a full-tendon transposition, the muscle is reattached parallel to the lateral border of the paralytic muscle rather than parallel to the insertion. The advantages and disadvantages are the same as those of a full-tendon transposition (Fig. 5–6).

The Hummelsheim procedure consists of taking half of the adjacent rectus and relocating it to the insertional border of the paralytic muscle (Fig. 5–7). The major advantages of this procedure are preservation of anterior ciliary arteries, simplicity of technique, and the ability to combine the procedure with a resection-recession of the transposed tendons for a complicated horizontal and vertical deviation. The disadvantages include splitting of the rectus, which causes hemorrhage and possible fibrosis, and complicated reoperations.

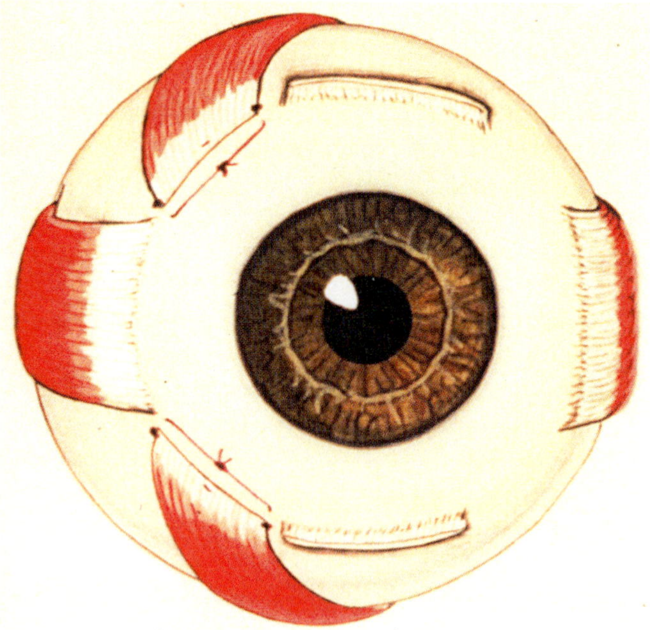

Figure 5–3. Full-tendon transposition. Appearance of full-tendon transposition for paralytic lateral rectus. Note that relative distances from the insertion to the limbus have been preserved, but the insertions have been displaced laterally to lie immediately adjacent to the lateral rectus insertion. The same procedure can be used for any isolated weakness of the rectus muscle.

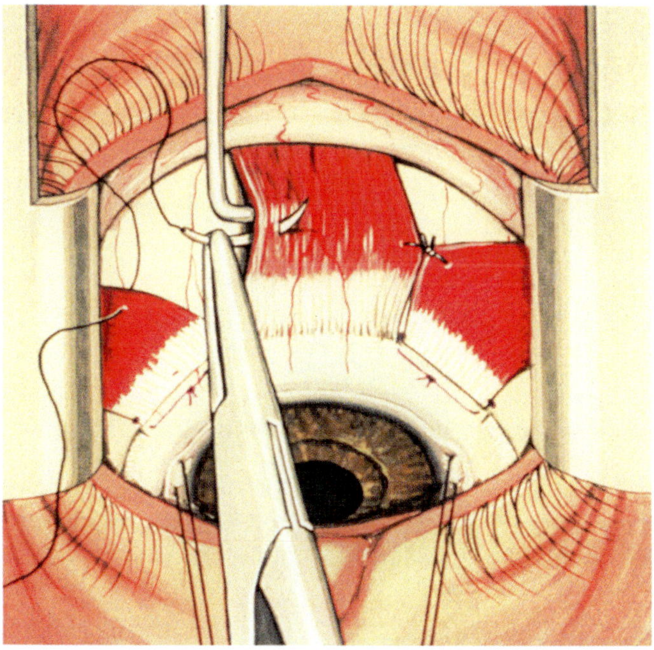

Figure 5–4. Buckley procedure. The effect of transposition can be further enhanced by suturing the border of the transposed muscles to the paralytic muscle. Nonabsorbable suture is placed 6.0 to 8.0 mm from the insertion along the lateral border of the transposed muscle. The suture is passed through the border of the paralytic muscle and tied loosely. The procedure is repeated for the other transposed muscle.

SIXTH NERVE PALSY

A sixth nerve (abducens) palsy is the most common acquired oculomotor palsy. Clinically, it presents as paralysis of the ipsilateral lateral rectus, which results in an abduction deficit toward the side of the lesion (esotropia) and horizontal

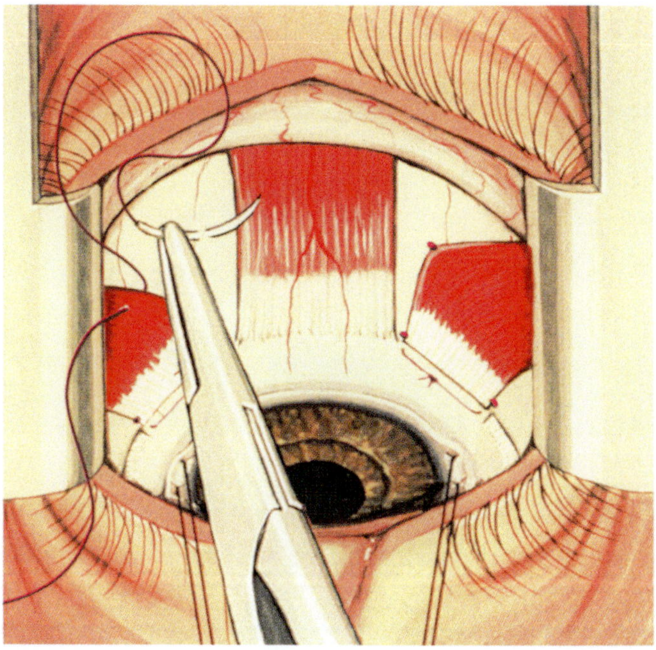

Figure 5–5. Foster suture. The full-tendon transposition procedure can be further enhanced by suturing the transposed muscle to the sclera 6.0 to 8.0 mm posterior to where the insertion is attached. This can be be done in a fashion similar to that of fadenoperation. Nonabsorbable suture is advised.

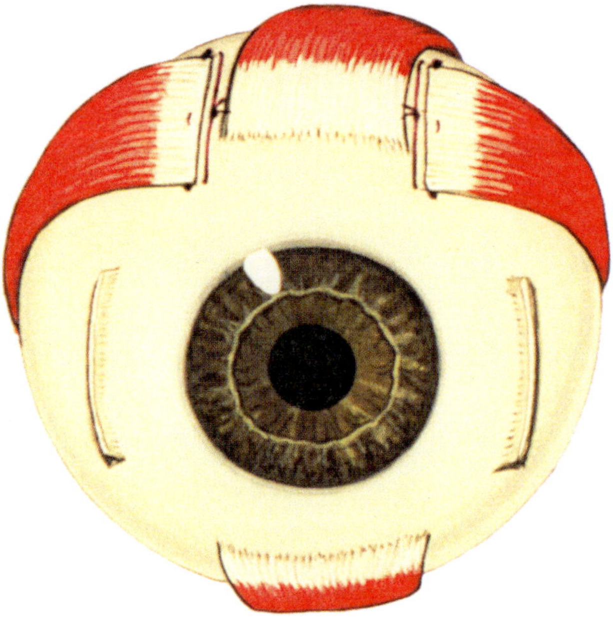

Figure 5–6. Knapp procedure. The entire rectus is transplanted to the paralytic muscle. Unlike full-tendon transposition, the muscle is reattached with an insertion parallel to the lateral border of the paralytic muscle rather than parallel to the limbus.

diplopia. In most patients, an acute acquired esotropia is due to a sixth nerve palsy. However, a thorough ophthalmic and neuro-ophthalmic evaluation is necessary to eliminate the other causes of abduction deficits (Table 5–1).

Patients with an acute-onset sixth nerve palsy complain of horizontal diplopia worse at distance than at near and worse on right or left gaze. They often have a

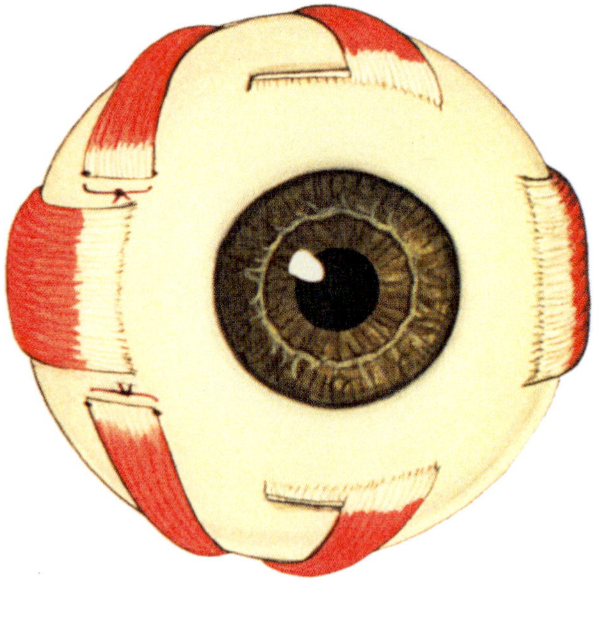

Figure 5–7. Hummelsheim procedure. Half of the adjacent rectus is relocated to the insertional border of the paralytic muscle. Advantages include preservation of anterior ciliary arteries. Disadvantages include extensive rectus manipulation and complicated reoperations.

Table 5–1 Causes of Abduction Deficits

Sixth nerve palsy
Graves' myopathy (fibrotic medial rectus)
Myasthenia gravis
Orbital inflammatory pseudotumor
Orbital trauma (medial rectus entrapment)
Congenital defects (Duane syndrome, Möbius syndrome)
Convergence spasm

head turn toward the side of the palsy. On examination, there is an obvious decrease in abduction of the involved eye with a large esotropia in the field of gaze of the paretic lateral rectus. Occasionally, a vertical deviation may also be present, although this is usually less than 5 prism diopters (Δ). A larger vertical deviation should alert the examiner to an accompanying fourth nerve palsy (which may be due to a cavernous sinus lesion) or a skew deviation, indicating brain stem dysfunction.

Ocular motility measurements should include the preferred position, the forced primary position, and lateral-gaze measurements. In general, measurements should be performed with the nonparalytic eye fixating. Measurements are much larger when the paralytic eye is fixating (secondary deviation). In addition to assessing ocular rotations, forced duction testing may be necessary to determine whether the decreased abduction is due solely to a paresis of the lateral rectus or whether there is some contracture of the medial rectus. This is especially important in long-standing sixth nerve palsies, since the medial rectus is almost always tight. Identifying a tight medial rectus is important in determining the appropriate surgical strategy.

Nonsurgical Treatment. The use of botulinum in acute sixth nerve palsies is controversial. The concept is that injecting botulinum toxin into the medial rectus will prevent contracture and, at the same time, create some areas of single binocular vision while the sixth nerve function recovers. Since the duration of the botulinum toxin effect is approximately the same as the recovery time for most sixth nerve palsies, the patient maintains a centered field of single binocular vision that widens as the palsy and the toxin effect on the medical rectus muscle resolve. The usefulness of botulinum toxin in preventing the development of esotropia from contracture has not been proven. Botulinum toxin has been shown to be helpful in reducing the esotropia in cases of chronic sixth nerve palsy with residual abduction deficits and can be used in cases where surgery is contraindicated.

COMMENT

Gunter K. von Noorden, MD

Among the nonsurgical treatment options in patients with milder forms of paralytic strabismus in whom recovery can be expected or surgery is delayed for other reasons, we consider sector occlusion of spectacle lenses with semiopaque Scotch tape. This allows the patient to enjoy single binocular vision, except when looking in the direction(s) of the paretic muscle(s). For instance, it is helpful to occlude the lower segment of a spectacle lens in a patient with superior oblique paresis who has diplopia only in down gaze or the nasal segment of each lens in a patient with bilateral sixth nerve paresis.

Surgical Treatment. The vast majority of patients with sixth nerve palsy who recover function will do so within 4 to 6 months. If a residual esodeviation persists beyond 6 months, surgical treatment should be considered. The timing of the surgery depends on the clinical course. If the esodeviation appears to be worsening with time, then medial rectus contracture is a component and interventions may be considered sooner than 6 months. If, however, sixth nerve function has been improving, then delaying surgical intervention beyond 6 months is also indicated.

The surgical approach depends on the two factors outlined previously: *the residual muscle function and the field of greatest deviation.* In the case of a sixth nerve palsy, the involved muscle is the lateral rectus, the antagonist muscle is the ipsilateral medial rectus, and the yoke muscle is the contralateral medial rectus. Some combination of surgery on these three muscles, plus a transposition procedure in complete paralysis, are the surgical options. The following examples illustrate how to use the clinical assessment to design a successful surgical procedure.

Mild limitation. Figure 5–8 illustrates a patient with a mild left sixth nerve palsy. There is a small esotropia in the primary position, which becomes worse on left gaze. The patient is orthophoric on right gaze. In this situation, the abduction force of the left lateral rectus is relatively good. A recession of the left medial rectus, alone or in combination with a resection of the left lateral rectus, will return the eyes to orthophoria in the primary position and will improve the esodeviation on left gaze. However, an unwanted effect will be an exotropia on right gaze (Fig. 5–8A). Depending on the amount of medial rectus recession or lateral rectus resection, this exodeviation can actually be quite large.

To minimize this lateral incomitance in a field where there was none previously, an alternative approach is to recess the medial rectus on the contralateral eye (Fig. 5–8B). This matches the weakness in the left eye with a similar weakness in the same field of gaze on the right. The patient is still orthophoric in the primary position, and there is less likely to be a significant exodeviation on right gaze. This concept of creating a matching weakness in the uninvolved eye is fundamental to achieving a wide range of single binocular vision in patients with paralytic strabismus.

Moderate limitation. The treatment of a moderate paresis requires combination surgery. First, a strengthening procedure on the paretic muscle is necessary. As an example, in a left sixth nerve palsy, the left lateral rectus must be resected. There also must be a weakening procedure on either the yoke (left medial rectus) or the antagonist muscle (right medial rectus). Which muscle is selected depends on the

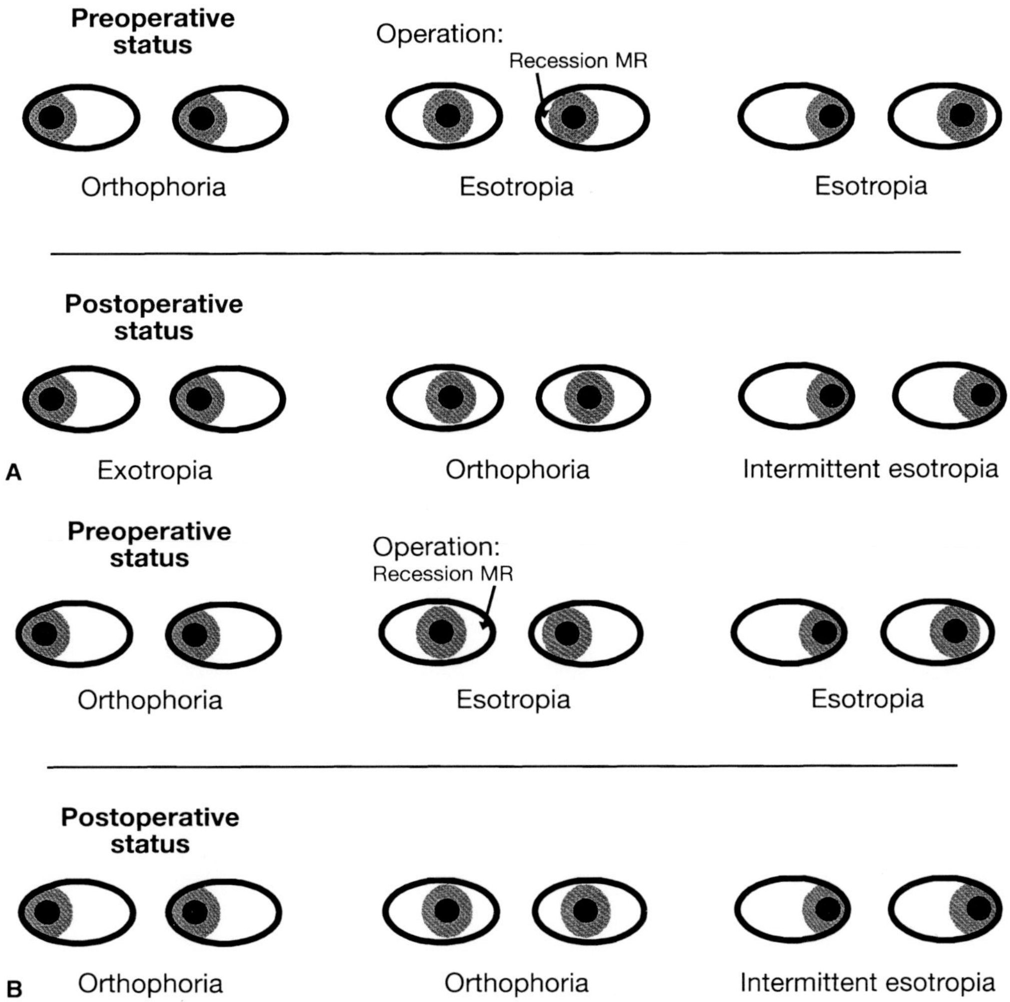

Figure 5–8. Left sixth nerve palsy (mild defect). (*A*) This patient has small-angle esotropia in the primary position, which increases on left gaze, and is orthophoric on right gaze. An operation on the ipsilateral medial rectus (MR) will result in alignment in primary position and improvement on left gaze but will create exotropia on right gaze. (*B*) This patient has mild left sixth nerve palsy similar to that in A. A surgical option is to recess the contralateral yoke MR. This aligns the eyes in primary position and improves alignment on left gaze without creating exotropia on right gaze.

direction in which deviation is greatest and the amount of deviation present on the opposite lateral gaze (right gaze).

If the deviation is somewhat comitant and there is a moderate esotropia on right gaze, then a recession of the antagonist left medial rectus will yield a satisfactory result. However, if the field of greatest deviation is in the direction of the involved muscle and there is little or no esotropia on right gaze, a recession of the antagonist left medial rectus will result in an exotropia on right gaze. An alternative operation, which will reduce the likelihood of this exotropia, is to recess the medial rectus of the right eye. This will limit the movement of the right eye on left gaze, balancing forces in that direction while reducing the likelihood of developing a significant exotropia on right gaze.

Consideration must be given to the possibility that no matter which medial rectus is recessed, an exodeviation will be created on right gaze. If this seems likely, a right lateral rectus recession can be performed either at the time of the original surgery or as a second procedure. When performed at the time of the original surgery, it allows for the optimal recession of the right medial rectus without the concern about creating an exodeviation on right gaze. The importance of avoiding the creation of an exodeviation in the one field of gaze where the patient was previously seeing single cannot be overemphasized.

Severe limitation. If there is no lateral rectus muscle function, then some form of alternative force must be created. There are two options:

1. The first is a large resection of the involved lateral rectus. This will tether the eye over in the field of action of this muscle. It will not increase the force generated in that direction, nor will it have much effect other than changing the resting position of the eye. This may be useful in those situations where transposition procedures cannot be performed. The best outcome in this situation is to center the eye with some movement medially and laterally.
2. The alternative is to perform a muscle transposition procedure.

In addition to providing an alternate force with the transposition or resection, the surgeon needs to weaken the overacting yoke medial rectus. Experience has shown that if full abduction can not be achieved then an esodeviation will usually persist on lateral gaze. A weakening procedure of the contralateral medial rectus will help reduce this esotropia.

If the ipsilateral medial rectus is contracted or tight, then a small recession of this muscle is also necessary to allow lateral movement of the eye. The presence of a restriction should be assessed at the time of the transposition procedure. To minimize the chances of anterior segment ischemia, the ipsilateral medial rectus usually is not recessed at the same time as the transposition procedure. Since reducing this restriction is necessary to maximize the effect of the transposition procedure.

COMMENT

Gunter K. von Noorden, MD

When planning a transposition for sixth nerve palsy with ipsilateral medial rectus contracture in patients at risk for anterior segment ischemia, I would perform the medial rectus recession first rather than the transposition. The reason is that a transposition is doomed to failure unless an opposing tight muscle is first released.

Injecting botulinum toxin into the medial rectus at the time of transposition surgery been found to be beneficial in temporarily weakening the medial rectus. It can also be injected prior to the surgical procedure, both as a clinical test to assess lateral rectus function and as preparation for the transposition procedure. Alternatively, botulinum toxin can be injected into the medial rectus several days after transposition surgery.

The major advantage of using botulinum toxin in this setting is to increase the amount of outward rotation of the eye in the immediate postoperative period. As the tissue heals in the abducted state, a greater passive force vector can be achieved. The major disadvantage is the prolonged recovery time until the final outcome can be assessed. Botulinum toxin injections may, however, obviate the need for ipsilateral medial rectus recession surgery in the future (Fig. 5–9).

COMMENT

Michael X. Repka, MD

In full-tendon transposition for total sixth nerve palsy, I augment the inferior and superior rectus lateral transpositions with a Foster or posterior suture. I inject botulinum toxin at the first postoperative visit (about 3 days) if the patient is still esotropic. If I do not use the Foster suture, then I inject botulinum toxin, 5–10 units, into the ipsilateral medial rectus muscle.

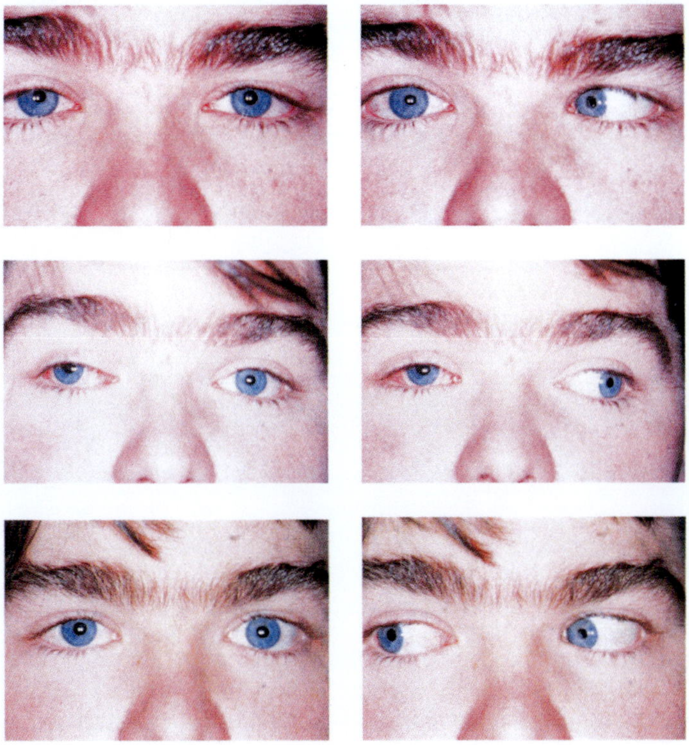

A

B

C

Figure 5–9. Complete right sixth nerve palsy. (*A*) Note the absent abduction of the right eye. (*B*) The patient has undergone a transposition procedure of the right eye, with botulinum toxin into medial rectus on the right. Note the mild ptosis from the botulinum toxin. There is also complete lack of adduction of the right eye. (C) The patient 6 months after botulinum toxin injection and full-tendon transposition of the right eye. Note the large degree of abduction. The patient has mild residual esotropia on extreme right gaze.

Occasionally, patients develop an exodeviation, especially on contralateral gaze. This is a result of the restriction created by the transposition surgery or the medial rectus recession. The exodeviation can be improved or eliminated by a large recession of the contralateral lateral rectus. If the eyes are straight in the primary position and the exodeviation is present only on lateral gaze, then a fadenoperation on the lateral rectus or a lateral rectus resection-recession operation can be used (Fig. 5–10).

In all of the above scenarios, weakening the contralateral medial rectus is helpful. While a recession is generally used, another effective technique is the fadenoperation. This procedure is especially useful in lateral rectus paresis and can provide an additional enhancement. In patients with mild limitation and a small deviation in the primary position, it can be combined with a recession. In more severe limi-

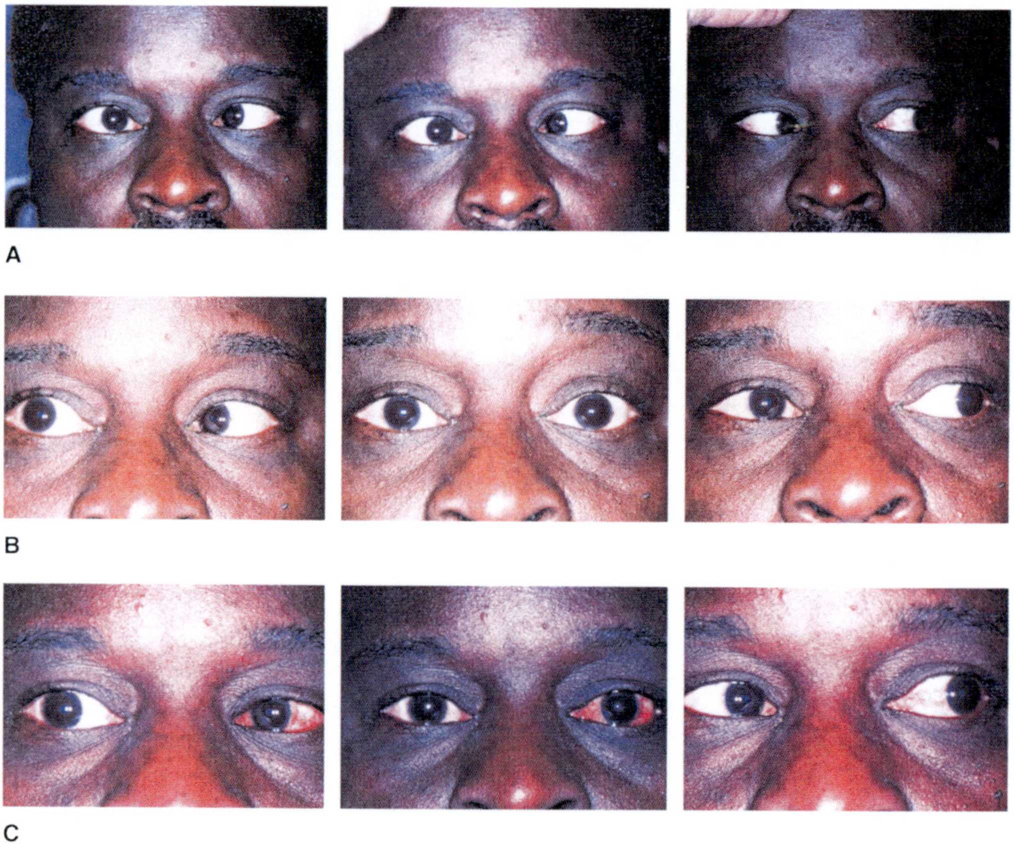

Figure 5–10. Complete right sixth nerve palsy. (*A*) Note the inability to abduct the right eye even to the midline. The patient had single binocular vision on extreme left gaze. (*B*) After full-tendon transposition, with recession of the medial rectus on the right, the patient is well aligned in primary position but continues to manifest esotropia on right gaze and has exotropia on left gaze. Weakening of the antagonist muscle is to be avoided unless it is restricted. (*C*) Resection with recession of the left lateral rectus was combined with a fadenoperation on the left medial rectus to eliminate lateral incomitance. The lateral rectus recession was performed on adjustable suture to maintain single vision in primary position.

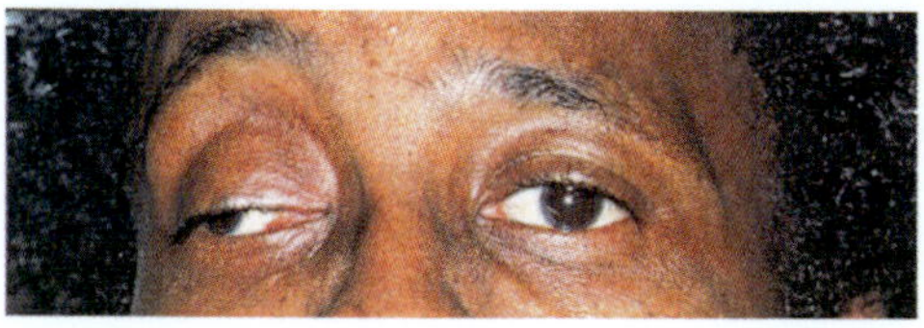

Figure 5–11. Complete third nerve palsy. Note the affected right eye is down and out. Ptosis and pupillary dilation are present.

tations, it can be used to expand the field of single binocular vision in the direction of the paralytic muscle. A major advantage is that it does not increase the risk of an exodeviation on contralateral gaze.

THIRD NERVE PALSIES

The third (oculomotor) nerve is responsible for elevation (superior rectus, inferior oblique), adduction (medial rectus), and depression (inferior rectus). It also provides innervation to the levator muscle, elevating the lid, and parasympathetic innervation to the pupil, causing constriction. A complete third nerve palsy results in ptosis, pupillary dilation, and the eye resting in the down and out position (Fig. 5–11).

Patients with an isolated third nerve palsy can present in a variety of ways (Table 5–2). Palsies that are caused by ischemia from microvascular disease tend to affect the deep oculomotor fibers and spare the peripheral pupillary fibers. The most common presentation of an ischemic third nerve palsy is the sudden onset of a painful ophthalmoplegia with normal-appearing pupils. The pain may be quite severe and may precede the ophthalmoplegia by days; alternatively, the pain may accompany the onset of ptosis or diplopia, which can be partial. Complete recovery usually occurs by 3 months. If the ophthalmoplegia does not improve after 6 to 8 weeks, neuroimaging should be considered. If ophthalmoplegia occurs with no pupil involvement and no pain, it is important to consider a muscle myopathy or a neuromuscular junction abnormality such as myasthenia gravis.

Aberrant regeneration of the third nerve may occur after traumatic or compressive injury, especially in traumatic third nerve palsies. This is manifested by paradoxical movements of the muscles and usually affects the lid and the pupil. A typical

Table 5–2 Isolated Third Nerve Palsy: Danger Ranking

Most ↑	Complete, plus pupil Probable aneurysm: internal carotid/posterior communicating artery
Dangerous	Complete, plus partial pupil Possible aneurysm: internal carotid/posterior cerebral artery, cavernous sinus
	Incomplete, pupil spared Rare aneurysm: superior cerebellar/posterior cerebral artery, cavernous sinus Mass: cavernous sinus, orbit
Least ↓	Complete, pupil spared Microvascular: diabetes, hypertension

presentation is elevation of the lid on attempted depression or adduction of the eye. These movements are due to miswiring of the nerves during the regeneration process. Aberrant regeneration never occurs with microvascular causes and is therefore not seen in third nerve palsies in diabetic patients. Primary aberrant regeneration without a preceding third nerve paresis is indicative of a tumor or aneurysm.

Nonsurgical Treatment.

Occlusion and prisms. In patients with total third nerve palsies, occlusion may be the only reasonable intervention. Patching of the involved eye is recommended to eliminate disorientation and pastpointing. Occlusion can also be used in partial third nerve palsies prior to consideration of surgical treatment or in those patients who are nonsurgical candidates because of associated neurologic disease or central disruption of fusion. In lieu of patching, Bangerder foils on glasses or occluder contact lenses can be used.

In patients with partial paralysis of the third nerve, it is sometimes possible to restore fusion with the use of Fresnel prisms. Since these patients often have a vertical and horizontal component, the goal is to restore fusion in the primary position and in down gaze. Fresnel prisms can be rotated to create both a horizontal and a vertical vector and should be placed on the paralytic eye if possible. Permanent prism glasses can be considered if the deviation is small and not amenable to strabismus surgery.

Botulinum toxin. The role of botulinum toxin is limited because of the number of extraocular muscles involved in third nerve paresis.

Surgical Treatment. Recovery from isolated third nerve palsy is usually rapid, with most patients showing some signs of improvement within 2 months. If no improvement occurs after 4 to 6 months, surgical intervention can be considered. The goals of strabismus surgery depend on the amount of residual third nerve function. It is usually not possible to regain normal ocular motility.

Near-total third nerve palsy. Patients with a near-total third nerve palsy usually have a large exotropia, with the eye either slightly hypertropic or slightly hypotropic (Fig. 5–12). There is very little elevation, depression, or adduction, and there is often contracture of the lateral rectus. The goal of surgery is to realign the eye in the primary position. These patients do not regain single binocular vision or, if they do, the window of single binocular vision is extremely small. With only two extraocular muscles functioning, it is impossible to regain much movement.

Since the superior and inferior rectus muscles are paretic, transposition procedures for the medial rectus paresis are ineffective. The only surgical strategy is to recess the tight lateral rectus and resect the paralytic medial rectus. Extremely large lateral rectus recessions need to be performed, and it is preferable not to do this with a hangback suture technique. The hangback technique allows the lateral rectus to creep forward, resulting in recurrence of the exotropia. The lateral rectus should be sutured to the eye 14.0 to 16.0 mm behind the insertion. At the same time, an extremely large (10.0 to 14.0 mm) medial rectus resection should be per-

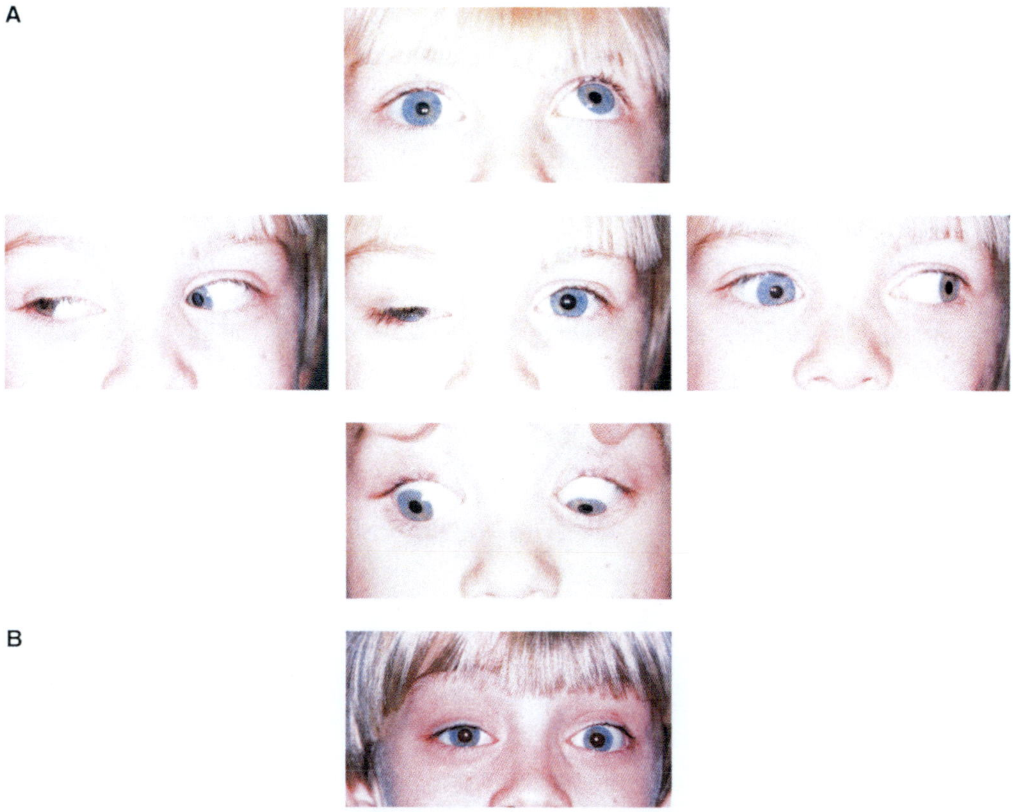

Figure 5–12. Third nerve palsy. (*A*) A child presents with total third nerve palsy of the right eye, which is down and out, and there is ptosis with aberrant regeneration. The medial rectus has moderate function; the superior and inferior rectus have poor function, with the inferior rectus being slightly stronger. (*B*) The patient underwent resection of the right medial rectus and recession of the left lateral rectus for exotropia and recession of the left superior rectus and fadenoperation on left inferior rectus for vertical deviation. Postoperatively, the patient had good primary-position alignment, with a fair range of coordinated movement horizontally and vertically. Note the improved lid position, which was achieved by taking advantage of the aberrant regeneration phenomenon.

formed. At the end of the surgery, there should be a significant restriction of abduction and the eye should be slightly esotropic. Failure to accomplish this will result in recurrence of the exotropia. Even with the lateral rectus recessed in this position, some abduction force will be preserved. This may be enough to give the patient a small range of single binocular vision.

Since the eye does not elevate or depress, no surgery on the vertical muscles is necessary unless there is a significant hypotropia or hypertropia. If there is a vertical deviation, it can be dealt with in one of two ways:

1. The resected medial rectus can be supraplaced or infraplaced in the appropriate direction to improve the vertical deviation; that is, if the eye is high, then the medial rectus would be resected and slightly infraplaced, and vice versa.
2. Alternatively, the vertical deviation can be improved by resecting the appropriate weak vertical rectus muscle to produce a tethering affect.

COMMENT
Marshall M. Parks, MD

My experience is that the eye is hypotropic due to a functioning fourth cranial nerve. This can be confirmed by the observation of incyclotorsion of the iris crypts of the exotropic involved eye as down gaze is attempted. In treating the total third nerve and its expected hypotropia, my surgical plan usually includes a tenotomy of the ipsilateral superior oblique. The tenotomy is not performed until after the large recession of the lateral rectus and resection of the medial rectus have allowed assessment of the adequacy of the intended correction of the exotropia, because transposition of the superior oblique tendon to the medial rectus is the trump card to further improve the residual exotropia if needed.

COMMENT
David A. Plager, MD

In total third nerve palsy with no adduction, the lateral rectus cannot be weakened too much or recessed too far. In such cases, including congenital total third nerve palsies, the lateral rectus can be disinserted from the globe and attached to the lateral orbital wall or (my preference) *extirpated* by dissecting around it far posteriorly to the Tenon's capsule penetration site, resecting as much muscle as can be reached and letting the residual stump retract through Tenon's capsule.Instead of a maximal resection of the medial rectus muscle, a passive adducting force is generated by disinserting the superior oblique tendon, resecting as necessary, and attaching it to the globe at the superior border of the medial rectus insertion (without taking the tendon out of the trochlea). This straightens the eye horizontally, albeit with minimal horizontal movement, and decreases the hypotropia by negating the infraduction normally supplied by the superior oblique.

COMMENT
Michael X. Repka, MD

I have begun disinserting the lateral rectus muscle and sewing it with a nonabsorbable suture to the lateral orbital wall 5.0 to 6.0 mm posterior to the lateral orbital rim. There is no way to achieve active adduction, but to hold the eye in primary position, a periosteal strip could be connected to the medial rectus insertion.

Many patients seem to tolerate the diplopia from a total third nerve palsy and are content to have the eye just "look better." However, some patients are bothered by intractable diplopia and need some sort of patch in order to function.

These patients need to be cautioned about undergoing surgery since preoperatively, the diplopic images are quite far apart and any attempt to align the eyes will bring these images closer together which may increase the patient's symptoms.

Most patients with complete third nerve palsy also have a ptosis. The ptosis should be addressed after ocular motility surgery. Full corrective repair is not possible due to the lack of Bell's phenomenon in these patients. A partial ptosis correction with a frontalis sling technique with a silicone rod can be performed, but care should be taken not to overcorrect, as exposure can be a significant problem. In those patients who have aberrant regeneration, tightening of the medial rectus with a corresponding weakening of the lateral rectus may increase innervation to the lid and improve the ptosis.

Partial third nerve palsy. Patients with a partial third nerve palsy can be approached with the same surgical principles used for sixth nerve palsies. These patients fall into two groups, those with primarily isolated muscle involvement and those with multiple muscle involvement:

1. *Isolated muscle involvement:* The goals of surgery in isolated muscle involvement are very similar to those for the treatment of sixth nerve palsies. The basic approach is to center the field of single binocular vision and make it as wide as possible. To accomplish this, surgery on the uninvolved eye is usually necessary; in particular, the yoke muscle of the paralytic muscle usually needs to be recessed.

   Table 5–3 illustrates the possible scenarios that might occur. As an example, the options for a patient with a right medial rectus weakness, due to either a third nerve palsy or an intranuclear ophthalmoplegia, are shown in Figure 5–13. If there is only mild medial rectus weakness and the field of greatest deviation is in the direction of the paralytic medial rectus, a recession of the contralateral lateral rectus is recommended. If the paresis is moderate, then a resect-recess operation on either eye would be appropriate. In severe limitations, alternate force needs to be created. This requires either a signifi-

Table 5–3 Isolated Muscle Paresis (Third Nerve Innervated)

Muscle	*Mild*	*Moderate*	*Severe*
MR	Recession yoke LR ±resection MR	Resection MR Recession LR	Transposition IR/SR Resection MR Recession yoke LR
SR	Resection SR or recession yoke IO	Resection SR Recession IR	Transposition MR/LR Recession contralateral SR
IR	Resection IR or recession yoke SO	Resection IR Recession SR	Transposition MR/LR Recession/fadenoperation contralateral IR
IO	Recession yoke SR	Recession SO Recession yoke SR	Recession SO Recession yoke SR

IO = inferior oblique; IR = inferior rectus; LR = lateral rectus; MR = medial rectus; SO = superior oblique; SR = superior rectus.

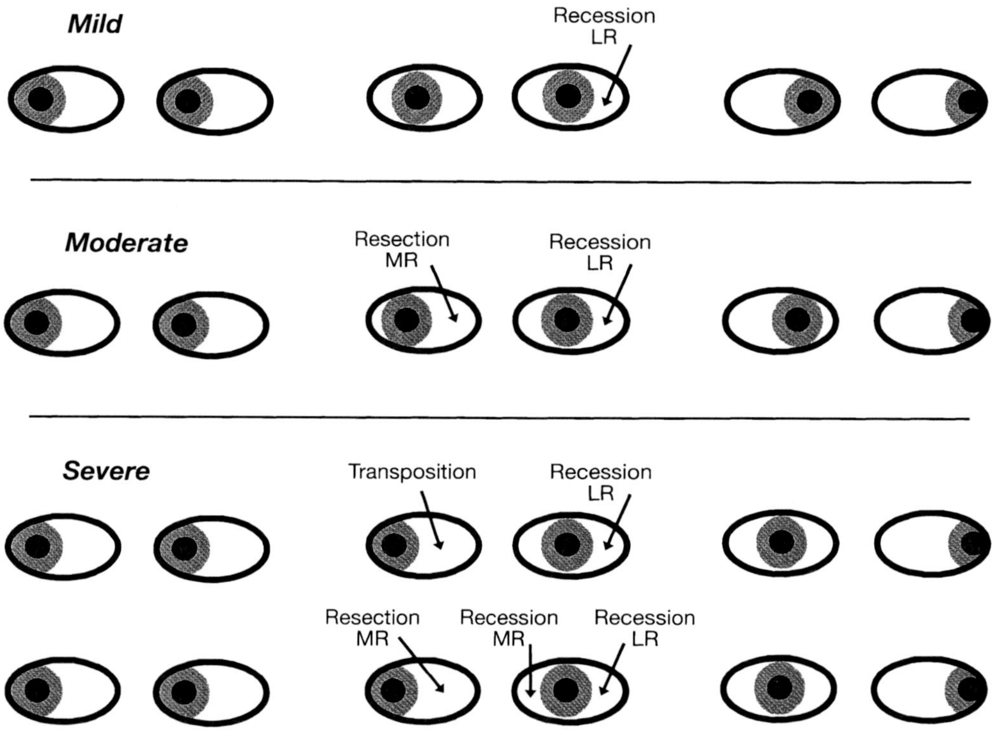

Figure 5–13. Isolated right medial rectus palsy. Mild weakness can be improved by recessing the yoke lateral rectus (LR). Moderate limitations require recession of the ipsilateral lateral rectus combined with a strengthening procedure on the weak medial rectus (MR). Severe limitations require some form of alternative force, either a transposition procedure or a large resection. The contralateral yoke also needs to be recessed. The contralateral medial rectus may need to be recessed for an induced esotropia on right gaze.

cant medial rectus resection or a transposition of the superior and inferior to the medial rectus insertion. Medial transpositions are less effective than lateral transpositions, and a small resection of the transposed muscles can be helpful. This by itself will not significantly improve the deviation in lateral gaze; a large recession of the contralateral lateral rectus will be necessary.

In general, some combination of resection of the involved muscle or a transpostion procedure to the paralytic muscle, plus a recession of the antagonist muscle and recession of the contralateral yoke muscle is needed. The selection of these muscles depends on the two fundamental principles of *residual muscle function* and *field of greatest deviation* (see Fig. 5–1). The surgical outcome may be modified by employing the adjustable suture technique.

Care should be exercised in recessing the antagonist muscle, especially in vertical deviations in third nerve palsies that appear to involve only an isolated muscle. Often, there is asymmetric involvement, with one of the vertical muscles more paretic than the other. A recession of the apparently normally functioning vertical muscle may result postoperatively in a more than anticipated underaction of this muscle. Recessing the *contralateral* yoke muscle will avoid this complication.

2. *Multiple muscle involvement:* In patients who have more than one paretic muscle, the outcome goals need to be altered, as it is usually impossible to obtain full function. Emphasis should be placed on aligning the eyes cen-

trally and in the down-gaze position. Alternative forces are usually necessary and will require either a transposition or a large resection.

Multiple muscle involvement can also be approached using the previously described concepts of muscle function and field of greatest deviation. Each muscle is assessed independently using these parameters, with the results combined to design a surgical approach. For example, Figure 5–14 illustrates the motility findings in a 65-year-old patient with a right third nerve palsy. The patient is unable to elevate and adduct the right eye. He has

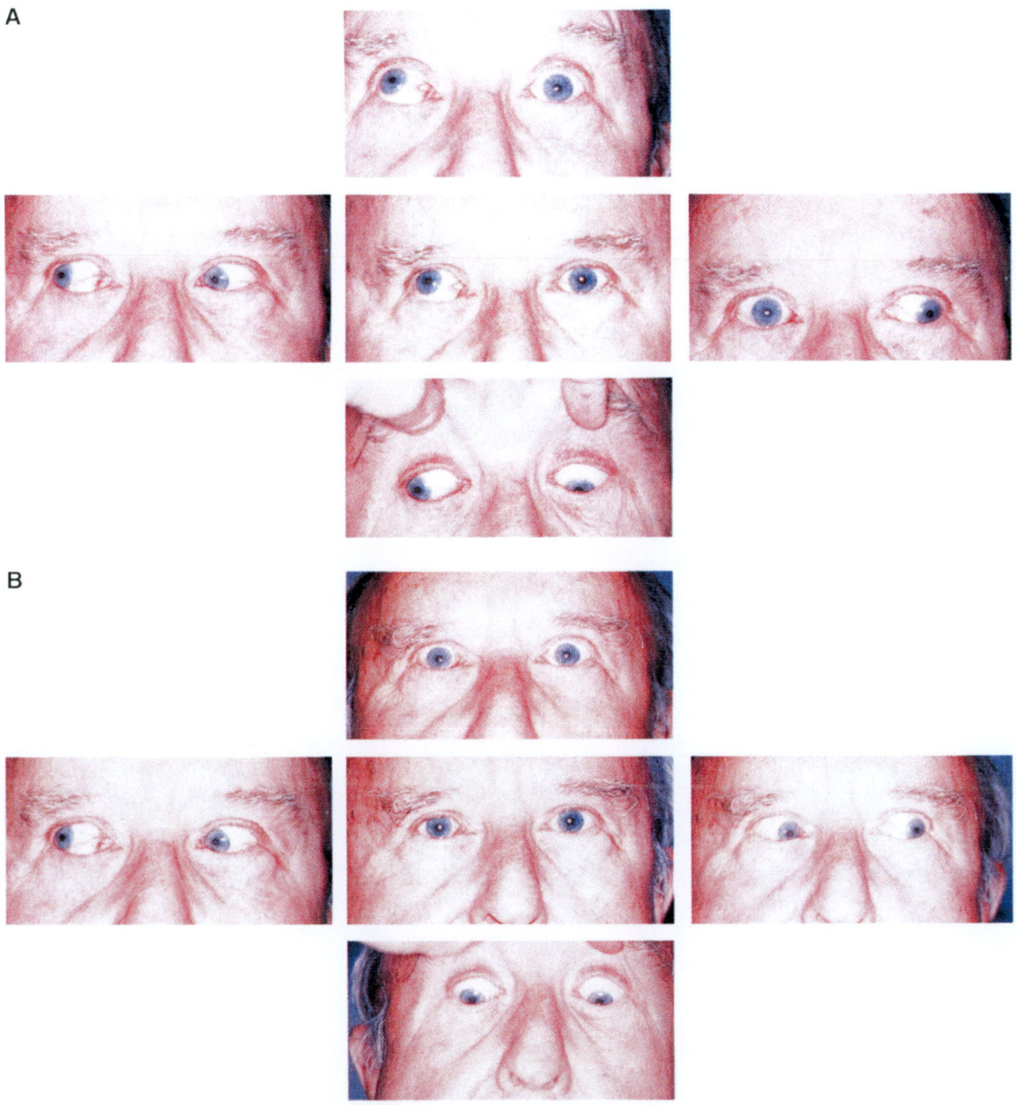

Figure 5–14. Right nuclear third nerve palsy. (*A*) Note the limitation of depression and adduction of the right eye and absent elevation of the left eye. The right third nerve nucleus supplies innervation to the left superior rectus. (*B*) To provide adducting and depressing forces, the right medial and right inferior rectus muscles were resected, allowing for single binocular vision in primary position, left gaze, and down gaze. A small esotropia was created in right gaze. Up gaze was limited in both eyes due to the paretic superior rectus on the left and the tight inferior rectus from resection on the right but did not bother the patient.

an exotropia that appears relatively similar in all horizontal-gaze positions and a marked right hypotropia.

As shown in Table 5–3, he will need an alternate force for the right superior rectus because there is no function, and a resection of the right medial rectus with either a right lateral rectus recession or a left lateral rectus recession. Since a transposition can be combined with a resect-recess procedure, the entire surgery can be performed on his right eye, involving only two of the rectus muscles. The medial rectus is resected and transposed superiorly to the medial border of the superior rectus, and the lateral rectus is transposed to the lateral border of the superior rectus and recessed with reference to the spiral of Tillaux. The resection-recession can actually be done with an adjustable suture technique if desired (Fig. 5–15).

COMMENT

Marshall M. Parks, MD

I have encountered poor results in adjusting the recess-resect measurements to simultaneously attempt correction of the horizontal component of the strabismus while doing the Knapp procedure. The side on which the resection is performed tends to pull the eye down when it turns toward that side and allows the eye to elevate when it turns toward the side of the muscle that received the recession procedure.

Other combinations of partially functioning muscles can be approached in the same manner (Fig. 5–16). The underlying general principles are always to improve rotation into the paretic muscle's field of action and to weaken yoke muscles.

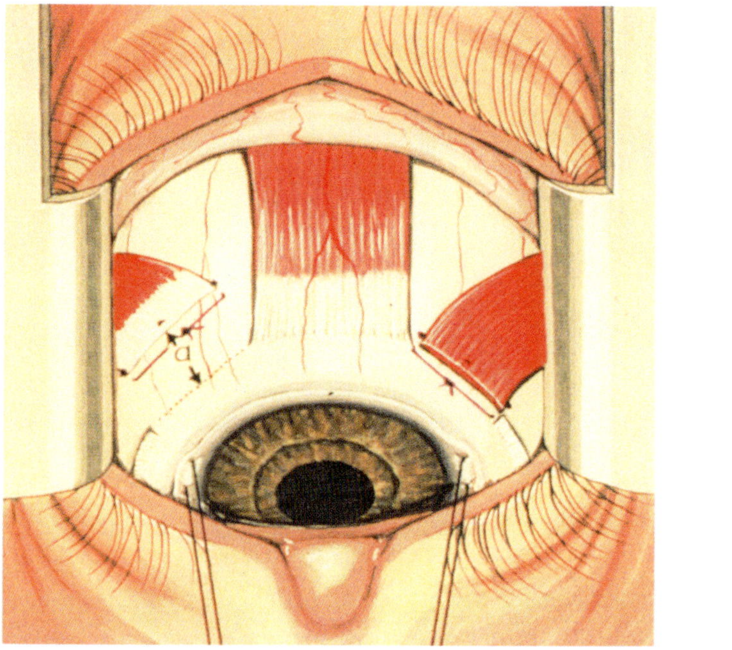

Figure 5–15. Full-tendon transposition can be combined with recession and resection of transposed muscles to address a secondary deviation. In this patient with a hypotropia in addition to lateral rectus palsy, the inferior rectus was recessed and the superior rectus was resected to correct hypotropia as part of the full-tendon transposition procedure for the esotropia. Recession was performed relative to the new insertion (dotted line) and was moved back at distance A in relation to it. The resected muscle was reattached at the new insertion adjacent to the lateral rectus.

A

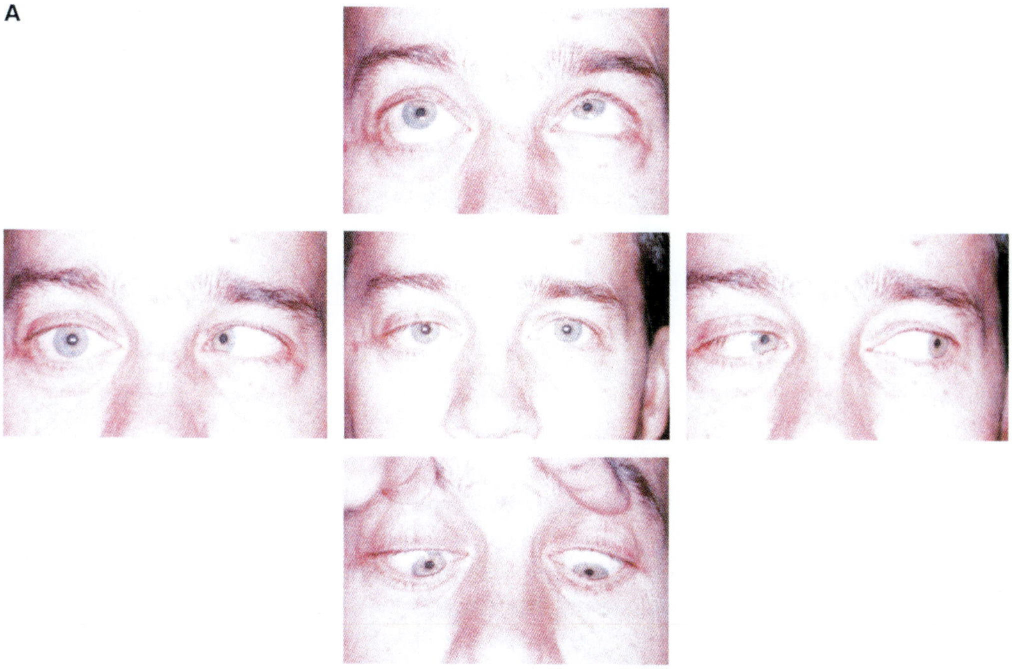

B

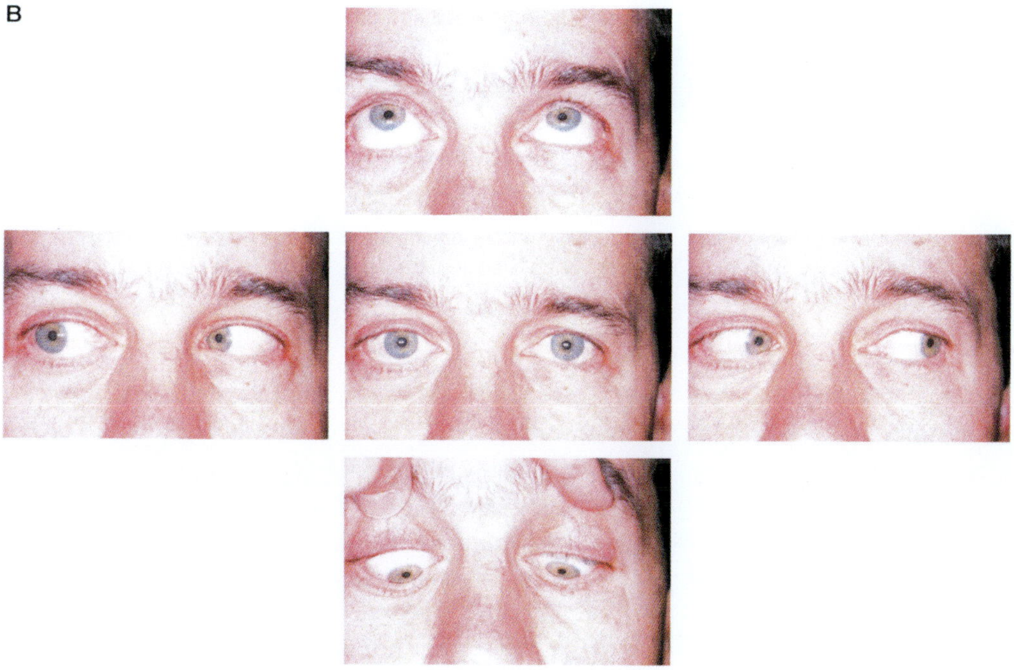

Figure 5–16. Right sixth and third nerve palsy. (*A*) The patient underwent orbital surgery of the right eye. There is combined weakness of the sixth and third nerves. Mild ptosis is present, with mild limitation of elevation and depression, as well as marked limitation of abduction. The patient has single binocular vision on extreme left gaze. (*B*) The surgical approach was broken down to take into account the separate muscle problems. For the abduction deficit, an alternate force needed to be created and a transposition procedure was performed. For the superior and inferior rectus weakness, the contralateral superior and inferior rectus muscles were equally recessed. The patient has a very wide area of single binocular vision but still has mild esotropia on right gaze. Lateral fadenoperation of the medial rectus on the left was performed.

Surgery on antagonist muscles can be used to enhance the resection effect, but this runs the risk of creating a deviation in a field where one did not previously exist.

Patients with aberrant regeneration and significant improvement in their ptosis on attempted adduction may benefit by a large medial rectus resection combined with a *contralateral* lateral rectus recession. Ptosis surgery should be deferred until after strabismus surgery has been performed.

COMMENT

David A. Plager, MD

The medial rectus in the involved eye may be operated on to reduce any exodeviation, but it is the lateral rectus recession (or medial rectus resection) in the *opposite* eye that calls Hering's law into action, increasing innervation to the medial rectus of the paretic eye, which in turn improves the ptosis via aberrant innervation of the eyelid.

DOUBLE ELEVATOR PALSY, OR MONOCULAR ELEVATION DEFICIENCY

The term *double elevator palsy* implies a paresis of both the inferior oblique and the superior rectus. This term has been used for any strabismus manifesting deficits in elevation in all positions of horizontal gaze. Since this motility pattern can be mimicked by inferior rectus restriction or isolated superior rectus paresis, the term *double elevator palsy* is misleading and is best replaced by *monocular elevation deficiency.*

Clinically, the patient presents with limitation of elevation in both adduction and abduction. The elevation deficit is often more pronounced in abduction than in the primary position and improves somewhat in adduction, in contrast to Brown syndrome (Fig. 5–17). There is a hypotropia of the involved eye that increases on up gaze. The patient will often use a chin-up position with fusion in down gaze. A pseudoptosis is often present in the primary position; however, an element of true ptosis is present in approximately 50% of patients (Fig. 5–18). In some patients, Bell's phenomenon is preserved, indicating a supranuclear defect. Since an inferior rectus restriction can have the appearance of a double elevator palsy, forced duction testing is necessary to plan a surgical treatment.

Surgical Treatment. Indications for treatment include a large vertical deviation in the primary position, with or without ptosis, and an abnormal head position with a gaze-down preference and a chin-up posture. If the inferior rectus on the involved side is restricted, then this muscle needs to be recessed (Fig. 5–19). This presents several problems. If the patient was fusing in down gaze, a recession of the tight inferior rectus will usually create an unwanted vertical deviation in down gaze postoperatively. To remedy this, a fadenoperation on the contralateral inferior rectus will be necessary (Fig. 5–20).

An alternative approach to avoid a significant down-gaze defect is to perform a smaller recession of the tight inferior rectus to free the restriction, combined with a recession of the contralateral superior rectus. Recessing the contralateral supe-

A

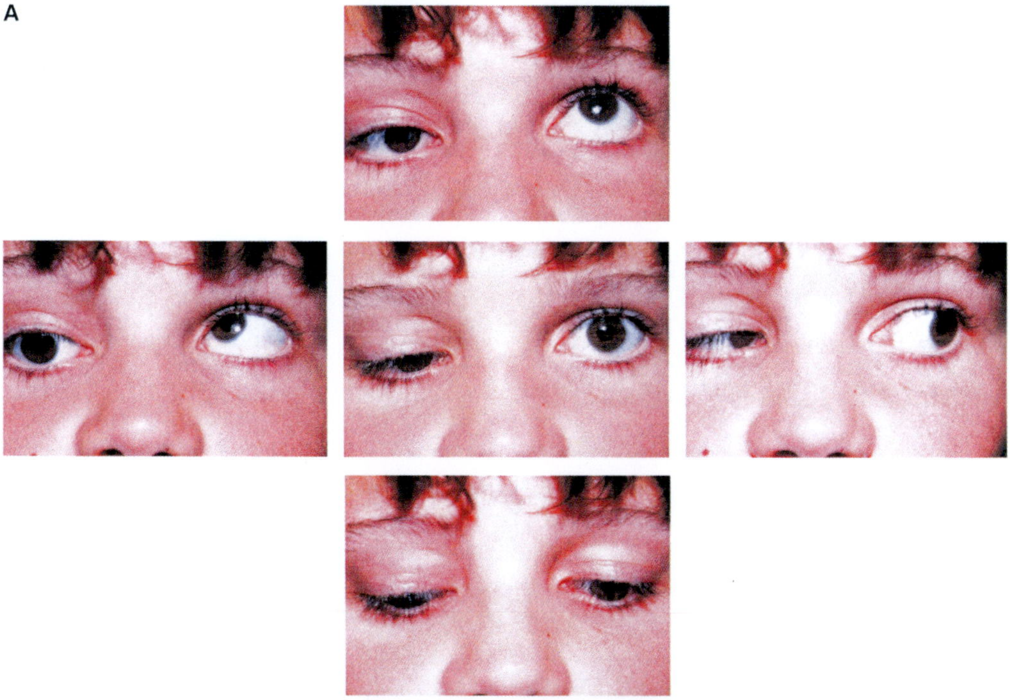

B

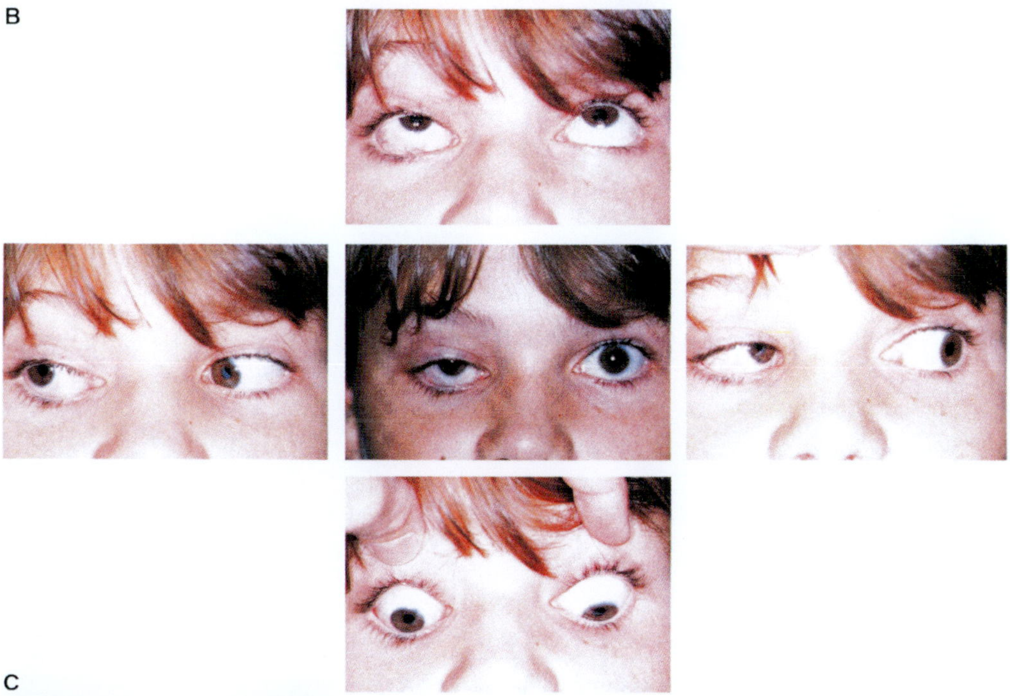

C

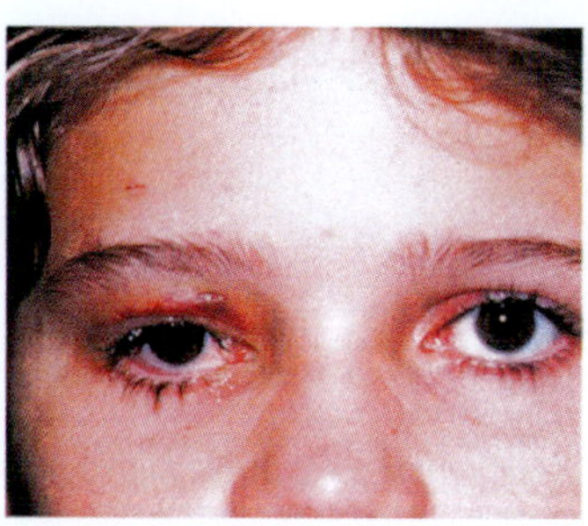

Figure 5–17. Right double elevator palsy. (*A*) Note the ptosis and inability to elevate the right eye in abduction and adduction. (*B*) The patient underwent medial and lateral rectus transposition superiorly. Note the markedly improved elevation of the right eye. There is a mild down-gaze weakness of the right eye. A left inferior rectus fadenoperation was required to eliminate this problem. Note the improvement in ptosis after strabismus surgery. (*C*) Residual ptosis was corrected with a frontalis sling.

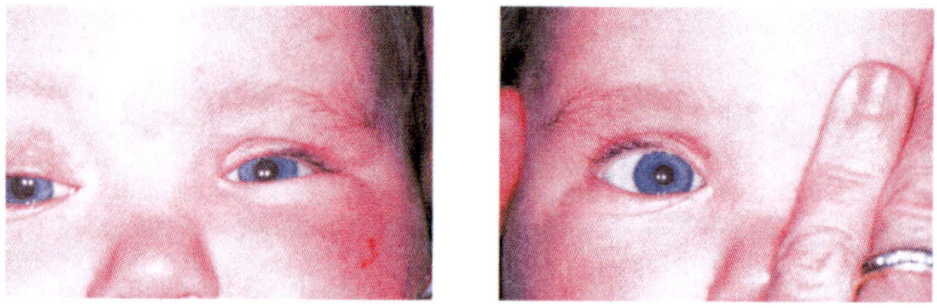

A B

Figure 5–18. Right double elevator palsy. (*A*) When the patient is fixating with the normal left eye, hypotropia and pseudoptosis affect the right eye. (*B*) When the patient is forced to fixate with the right eye, the ptosis resolves.

rior rectus will minimize the amount of inferior rectus recession required to obtain good alignment in the primary position.

Often, the inferior rectus is tight because of the paretic up-gaze situation. Simply freeing the inferior rectus will not give sufficient up-gaze force to align the eyes satisfactorily. In this circumstance, the addition of a transposition procedure may be indicated. Care must be taken not to overrecess the tight inferior rectus if this is combined with a transposition procedure, as a down-gaze defect can be created.

If no restriction is found or if, after inferior rectus recession, the eye still does not elevate, then a transposition procedure is necessary. The most popular transpositions for this condition are the Knapp procedure and a full-tendon transposition. Both are very effective in achieving balance in the primary position and allowing some upward movement of the eye. A transposition often has to be combined with a contralateral superior rectus recession to achieve a balanced result. Since it is difficult to predict how much elevation will be obtained, the contralateral superior rectus recession surgery usually is performed as a second procedure.

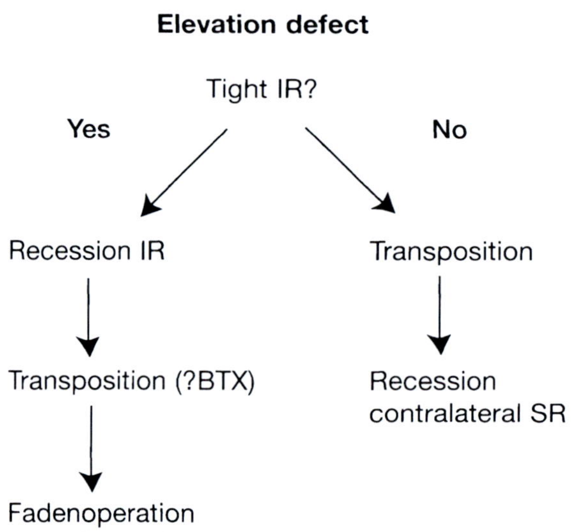

Figure 5–19. Double elevator palsy. The key deciding factor in devising a surgical strategy is whether the ipsilateral inferior rectus is contracted. If it is, recession of the inferior rectus must be performed. BTX = botulinum toxin; IR = inferior rectus; SR = superior rectus.

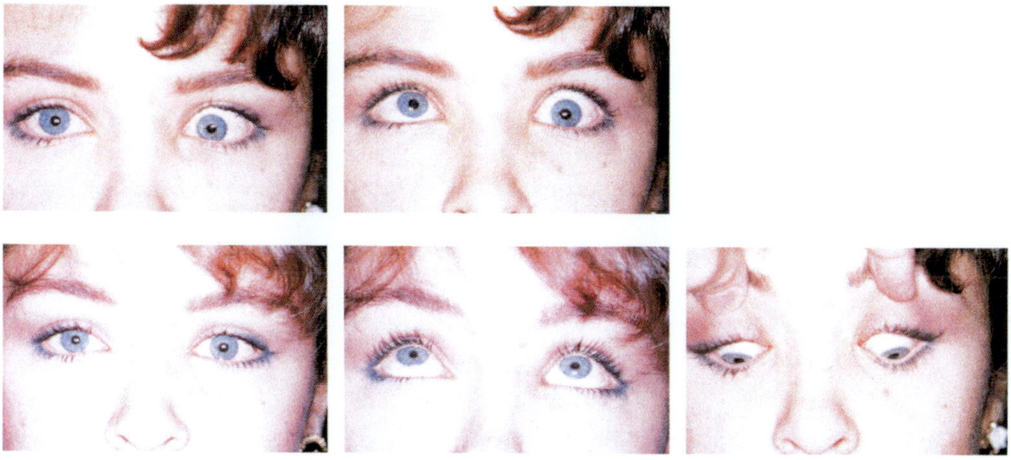

A

B

Figure 5–20. Double elevator palsy secondary to a restricted inferior rectus on the left. (*A*) Note the marked inability to elevate the left eye and the lid retraction on the left. (*B*) The patient underwent left inferior rectus recession and right inferior rectus fadenoperation. Note the markedly improved elevation of the left eye. The fadenoperation was a secondary procedure for surgically induced left hyperdeviation on down gaze. Note also the improvement in lid retraction.

Occasionally, the transposition procedure will be effective in aligning the eyes in the primary position, but it will cause a slight defect in depression through superior restriction. A fadenoperation on the contralateral inferior rectus may be necessary to restore alignment in the down-gaze position.

COMMENT

Marshall M. Parks, MD

Double elevator palsy, in my experience, is usually associated with exotropia. So common is this association that I have told students it is my dictum to correct the hypotropia on the palsied eye (Knapp procedure plus inferior rectus recession if the muscle is tight on traction testing) and to correct the exotropia by operating on the other eye.

INTERNUCLEAR OPHTHALMOPLEGIA

The medial longitudinal fasciculi (MLF) are paired nerve fiber tracts that function primarily as a connection between the pontine horizontal-gaze center and the vertical-gaze centers in the rostral midbrain. They also extend below the pons into the spinal cord. The MLF are located in the dorsal aspect of the median midbrain adjacent to the aqueduct. This pathway is particularly important because it connects the contralateral horizontal-gaze center with the ipsilateral medial rectus subnucleus, which provides eye coordination on lateral gaze. A lesion in this pathway will cause an adduction defect on the side of the lesion, with abducting nystagmus of the other eye, that is, internuclear ophthalmoplegia (INO). This can be unilateral or bilateral and is typically caused by a demyelinating plaque in younger patients or microvascular disease in older patients.

Table 5–4 Internuclear Ophthalmoplegia

	Involved Eye	Contralateral Eye
Unilateral		
Mild		Recession LR ±Recession MR
Moderate	Resection MR	Recession LR Recession MR
Severe	Resection MR	Recession LR Recession MR (?Fadenoperation)
Bilateral		
Mild	Recession LR OU	
Moderate	Resection MR OU	
Severe	Resection MR OU Recession LR OU	

LR = lateral rectus; MR = medial rectus; OU = both eyes (oculi uterque).

The typical presentation is acute onset of diplopia, mainly on horizontal gaze. Clinically, there is a unilateral or bilateral adduction defect that can range from very mild to complete inability to move past the midline. On extreme lateral gaze, the abducting eye may manifest a jerk nystagmus, with the fast component in the direction of gaze. A right INO would have decreased adduction of the right eye on left gaze, with the left eye manifesting a left jerk nystagmus on extreme left gaze. This abducting eye nystagmus can be seen in any situation where adduction of the contralateral eye is impaired and is not a consequence of the neurologic defect. The patient is usually orthophoric in the primary position, since tonic innervation is still present to the medial rectus. Convergence, which is mediated by another pathway, is usually intact. In rostral bilateral MLF lesions that interrupt the medial rectus subnucleus, an exotropia may occur. This is termed the *WEBINO* (*w*all-*e*yed *b*ilateral *in*ter*n*uclear *o*phthalmoplegia) *syndrome*. Magnetic resonance imaging (MRI) often demonstrates the lesion in the midbrain.

Surgical Treatment. Most patients with INO improve spontaneously, with symptoms resolving in 4 to 6 weeks. Occasionally, a persistent defect requires intervention. This condition behaves very much like other types of paralytic strabismus, and the same principles can be applied. The biggest obstacle is that transpositions, the mainstay of single paretic muscle treatment, are not as effective for the medial rectus as they are for other rectus muscles. This is because of the angle of muscle direction, which is straight posterior for the medial rectus and angled for the rest. Therefore, resections are substituted to increase medial rectus function and are used in combination with contralateral medical and lateral rectus recessions (Table 5–4).

The larger the primary-position exotropia, the more the involved medial rectus must be resected, as opposed to contralateral lateral rectus recession. The amount of resection is limited by the primary-position deviation. If this deviation is minimal, then either a recession or a fadenoperation of the contralateral medial rectus will need to be performed to avoid creating an esotropia in primary and opposite lateral gaze positions (Fig. 5–21).

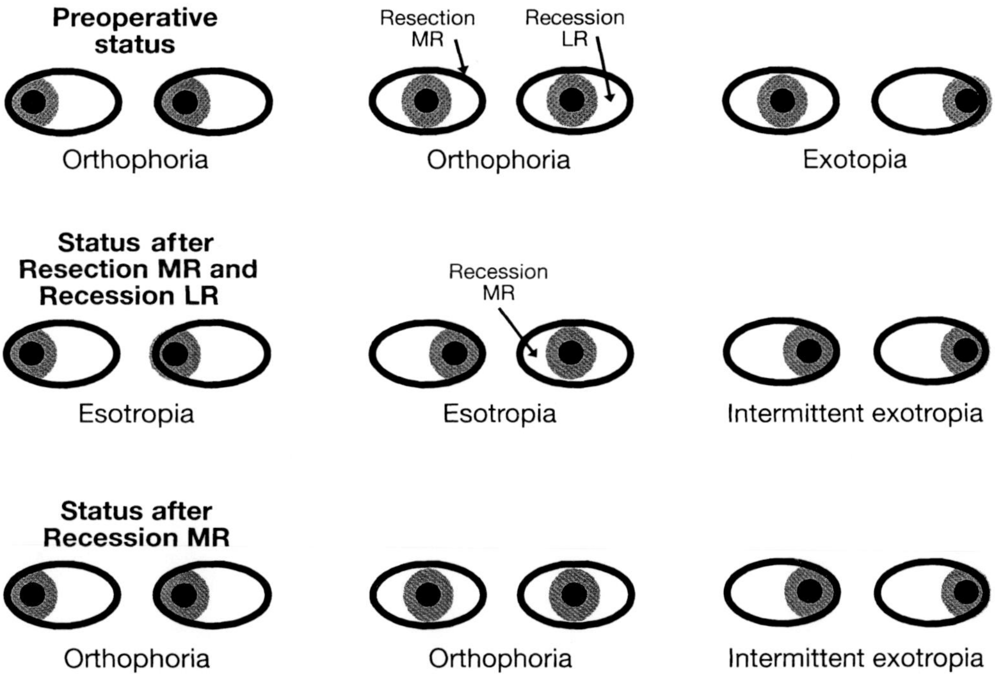

Figure 5–21. Internuclear ophthalmoplegia (INO). Severe right INO with large exodeviation on left gaze. To improve medial rectus function, resection of the right medial rectus (MR) must be performed. When this is combined with recession of left lateral rectus (LR), the large exodeviation on left gaze can be eliminated. However, this usually results in esotropia in the primary position. This can be improved by medial rectus recession or fadenoperation on the left. Ideally, this surgery can be done in a single operation.

Bilateral INO with a large exotropia can be treated with bilateral medial rectus resections alone unless a very large exotropia is present in the primary position. Even then, improving medial rectus function rather than weakening the lateral rectus is advisable to increase adduction forces.

OCULAR MYASTHENIA

A combined paresis–restriction condition, ocular myasthenia is a sequela of myasthenia gravis, an autoimmune neuromuscular disorder that is due to a defect in nerve-to-muscle transmission at the neuromuscular junction. Antibodies to muscle receptors block the neuronal signal, thereby weakening the muscle's response. If the extraocular muscles are involved, strabismus, which is very similar in character to that seen with cranial nerve palsy, results.

Clinically, myasthenia can masquerade as any of the oculomotor cranial nerve palsies, most commonly third and sixth. The patient presents with a variable strabismus that can involve one or both eyes. The presence of ptosis is a strong clue that myasthenia may be the cause. The condition usually worsens without treatment, and eventually both eyes show limited movement in all directions. Myas-

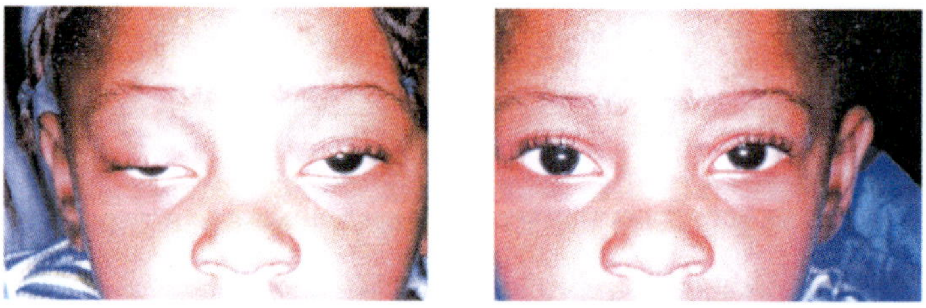

A B

Figure 5–22. Ocular myasthenia. (*A*) Note the asymmetric ptosis with exotropia. (*B*) Physostigmine was given intramuscularly, and an examination was performed 15 minutes later. Note the marked improvement in bilateral ptosis and exotropia.

thenia will remain purely ocular in only 20% of patients, with the majority eventually developing systemic signs and symptoms.

The key clinical features are ptosis and variable strabismus. These can often be detected during the examination, as the motility measurements keep changing from moment to moment. Special care should be taken to assess medial rectus, inferior rectus, and superior oblique function, as these are the muscles most commonly involved.

Pharmacologic testing with anticholinesterases is the standard initial test. Edrophonium (Tensilon) is injected intravenously, up to 10 mg in adults and 0.15 mg/kg in children. A positive response occurs within a minute and may be fleeting. Edrophonium can cause cholinergic side effects, so atropine must be readily available. False-negative test results are common if ptosis is not present. Some patients are hypersensitive, and the standard dosage can worsen the clinical findings. Intramuscular prostigmine 1.5 mg mixed with atropine 0.4 mg in adults (0.04 mg/kg with atropine and 0.3 mg in children) can also be used (Fig. 5–22). The patient is examined 15 to 20 minutes later. This is especially advisable in young children, who normally do not tolerate an intravenous test. A positive acetylcholine receptor antibody assay is diagnostic for myasthenia. Unfortunately, the test is negative in more than half of ocular myasthenic patients.

Single fiber electromyographic testing of the facial muscles is the most sensitive test and may be positive when all other tests are negative. Computed tomography (CT) scanning of the chest may reveal a thymoma. A small group of patients may have a completely negative initial workup, but if suspicions remain high, subsequent evaluations should be considered.

Nonsurgical Treatment. The treatment of myasthenia is initially directed at reducing the neuromuscular blockade and increasing the neurotransmitter chemical. Corticosteroids inhibit receptor antibody production, and acetylcholinesterase inhibitors (Mestinon) provide more chemical to stimulate available sites. In some cases, thymectomy is required to reduce the immune response, and plasmapheresis has been found useful in severe situations. Even with maximum therapy, the extraocular symptoms may not resolve. Under these circumstances, strabismus surgery can be indicated.

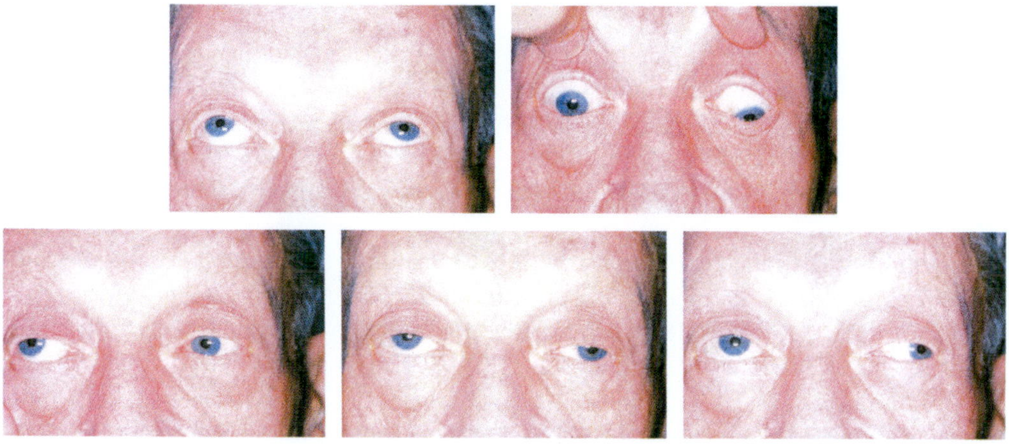

A

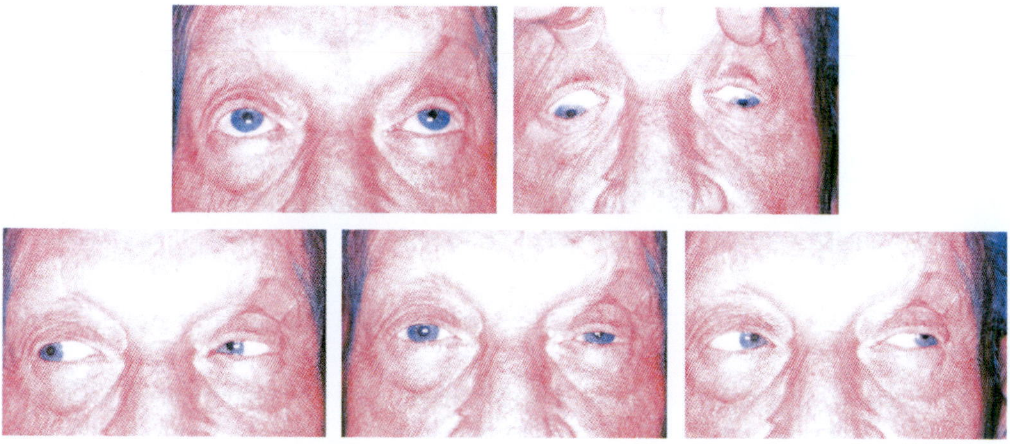

B

Figure 5–23. Long-standing ocular myasthenia. (*A*) Diplopia has persisted despite maximum medical therapy over many years. The patient has exotropia and hypertropia of the right eye. The right eye cannot be adducted and depressed. (*B*) The patient underwent resections of the medial and inferior rectus muscles of the right eye. There is residual mild exotropia on left gaze. The patient is orthophoric in primary and down-gaze positions. The result has been stable for more than 5 years.

Surgical Treatment. When strabismus surgery is contemplated in a patient with myasthenia, care should be taken to ensure that the condition is as stable as possible. If the measurements are highly variable, the surgical result will be difficult to predict. On the other hand, if, after prolonged treatment, a stable strabismus is present, then surgery can be attempted. This usually requires 6 to 12 months of observation. Even though ocular myasthenia is a form of paresis, the general rules for paralytic strabismus do not apply and have to be modified to take into account that all the extraocular muscles are often unequally involved.

In general, resections are more useful than recessions (Fig. 5–23). Resections strengthen muscle function and help balance opposing forces by making muscles equally strong. Since all the muscles are compromised to some extent, this approach retains as much function as possible. Recessions, while effective in eliminating a primary-gaze deviation, further weaken the muscle, increasing the overall dysfunction of the eye. Since, in most cases, movement is already limited, efforts should be directed at increasing rather than decreasing muscle function. Recessions cannot be completely abandoned since often there is a *restrictive component* to the strabismus. This is especially true if one muscle is severely impaired. In this situation, its antagonist will contract over time and must be loosened to improve ocular rotations. Forced duction testing is imperative to identify this possibility.

Rarely are transpositions helpful, since the adjacent muscles are also involved. Transposing weak muscles to assist has little advantage over resecting the involved muscle and may further weaken the transposed muscle's primary action, which was often only marginally acceptable before the surgery. Using adjustable sutures is helpful in obtaining the best alignment, since the effect of conventional amounts of surgery is unpredictable.

CHRONIC PROGRESSIVE EXTERNAL OPHTHALMOPLEGIA

Another combined paresis–restriction, chronic progressive external ophthalmoplegia (CPEO), is a disorder involving progressive ptosis and paralysis of extraocular muscles due to a mitochondrial abnormality. Initially, slowed saccades are present, with a variable ptosis. Involvement may be asymmetric, but it progresses to almost total ophthalmoplegia. However, patients often do not complain of diplopia. There is an accompanying weakness of the orbicularis oculi, but the pupil is not involved.

Chronic progressive external ophthalmoplegia may be associated with systemic abnormalities, including cardiac conduction defects (Kearns-Sayre syndrome), variable retinal pigmentary changes, and hearing impairment. Cardiac evaluation is essential, as complete heart block can result in sudden death. Demonstrable deletions of the mitochondrial genome are seen in more than 50% of patients, and ragged red fibers are found on special histologic staining of the muscle. Some patients also have involvement of other organs, such as the skin, endocrine glands, and skeleton (CPEO plus).

Ptosis is usually the first sign and may precede the ophthalmoplegia by years. It is usually bilateral but can be asymmetric early in the disease. Often, the ptosis results in a head tilt or chin-up position. The ophthalmoplegia is bilateral, with downward movements relatively intact compared to upward and horizontal movements, but most cases eventually proceed to complete ophthalmoplegia. There is usually a large-angle exotropia, with very limited movements in any direction. Cross cover testing is usually of very limited value in assessing the size of the deviation, but a modified Krimsky test can provide some information. Forced duction testing reveals only mild restriction, which is compatible with a chronic condition. Force generation is absent or subnormal. Muscle biopsy, typically of the leg muscles, often reveals the diagnosis. Differential diagnosis includes chronic myasthenia, progressive supranuclear palsy, parkinsonism, and oculopharyngeal dystrophy.

Surgical Treatment. Care must be taken in correcting the ptosis in this group of patients because the absent Bell's response puts them at increased risk for severe corneal exposure problems. Lid crutches and other less invasive procedures should be considered. If ptosis surgery is undertaken, brow suspensions, which can be titrated and even reversed, are advisable. Great care must be exercised not to overcorrect.

The goals of strabismus surgery are limited to placing the eyes in the primary position to help eliminate head positions and improve appearance. Limited binocular function can be achieved, but only in those patients with residual muscle function. As in other paretic situations, increasing the muscle force or tension is

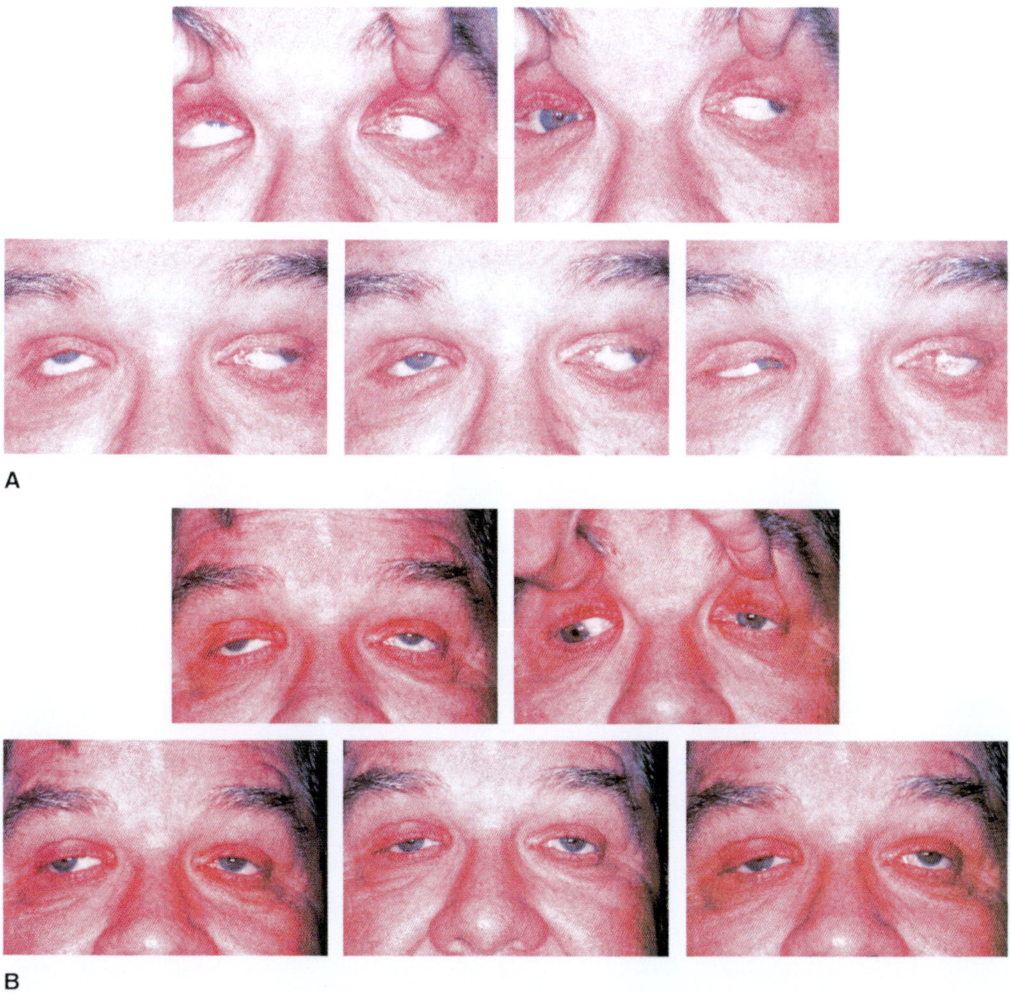

Figure 5–24. Long-standing chronic progressive external ophthalmoplegia. (*A*) The patient has bilateral ptosis and cannot move the eyes in all directions; down gaze is severely impaired. The patient has large-angle exotropia. Visual function is compromised because the eyes are elevated under the lids. (*B*) At the time of surgery, forced ductions were positive. Large medial rectus resection and lateral rectus recession of the left eye were performed. Postoperatively, the patient regained single binocular vision at distance but still had diplopia at near.

necessary to hold the eyes in position. Since none of the muscles has much function, tethering the eye is the most effective course and is accomplished with resections. Most patients have an exotropia and mild vertical deviation.

Extra-large medial rectus resections, combined with recession of the usually tight lateral rectus, are necessary (Fig. 5–24). These can be infraplaced if downgaze movement is desired. Undercorrections are common and can be avoided by ensuring that the patient is esotropic with a restricted medial rectus at the end of the procedure. Bilateral surgery is often necessary to achieve a satisfactory result.

Suggested Readings

Acheson JF, Elston JS, Lee JP, et al: Extraocular muscle surgery in myasthenia gravis. *Br J Ophthalmol* 1991; 75:232–235.

Buckley EG: Chemodenervation of extraocular muscles. In: Duane TD, ed: *Clinical Ophthalmology*, Vol 6. Philadelphia: JB Lippincott Co; 1993, Chapter 89.

Buckley EG: Fadenoperation (posterior fixation suture). In: Rosenbaum AL, Santiago AP, eds: Chapter 37 *Clinical Strabismus Management: Principles and Surgical Techniques.* Philadelphia: WB Saunders Co; 1999, 491–505.

Buckley EG, Meekins BB: Fadenoperation for the management of complicated incomitant vertical strabismus. *Am J Ophthalmol* 1988; 105:304–312.

Buckley EG, Shields M: *Strabismus and Glaucoma Surgery*, Vol 3. St Louis: CV Mosby Co; 1995.

Buckley EG, Townshend LM: A simple transposition procedure for complicated strabismus. *Am J Ophthalmol* 1991; 111:302–306.

Buncic JR: Sixth nerve palsy. In: Good WV, Hoyt CS, eds: *Strabismus Management.* Boston: Butterworth-Heinemann; 1996, 271–276.

Burke JP, Ruben JB, Scott WE: Vertical transposition of the horizontal recti (Knapp procedure) for the treatment of double elevator palsy: effectiveness and long term stability. *Br J Ophthalmol* 1992; 76:734–737.

Davidson JL, Rosenbaum AL, McCall LC: Strabismus surgery in patients with myasthenia. *J Pediatr Ophthalmol Strabismus* 1993; 30:292–295.

Foster RS: Vertical muscle transposition augmented with lateral fixation. *J Am Assoc Pediatr Ophthalmol Strabismus* 1997; 1:20–30.

Helveston EM: *Surgical Management of Strabismus: An Atlas of Strabismus Surgery*, 4th ed. St Louis: CV Mosby Co; 1993, 291–302.

Kushner BJ: Management of diplopia limited to down gaze. *Arch Ophthalmol* 1995; 113:1426–1430.

Metz HS: Twentieth annual Frank Costenbader Lecture: muscle transposition surgery. *J Pediatr Ophthalmol Strabismus* 1993; 30:346–353.

Rosenbaum AL: Adjustable vertical rectus muscle transposition surgery. *Arch Ophthalmol* 1991; 109:1346–1352.

Wallace DK, Sprunger DT, Helveston EM, et al: Surgical management of strabismus associated with chronic progressive external ophthalmoplegia. *Ophthalmology* 1997; 104: 695–700.

6

Restrictive Strabismus

EDWARD G. BUCKLEY

Treating strabismus secondary to a restriction is challenging because both the muscle and the surrounding tissue are involved. Since the cause in most cases is multifactorial, the treatment options are often complex and unpredictable. The preoperative evaluation should include an assessment of the degree of restriction (forced duction), muscle function (force generation), and the condition of the surrounding tissue.

PATIENT EVALUATION

The most important information needed to plan the surgical intervention is the amount of restriction. This is easily assessed by performing a forced duction test, which can be done either at the time of the initial evaluation in the office or in the operating room just prior to beginning the surgical procedure. During the test, it is important to determine the amount of limitation in *both* directions for each of the involved muscles. For example, in a patient with a blowout fracture of the floor of the orbit with involvement of the inferior rectus, both elevation and depression must be evaluated. In such situations, there can be limitations in up gaze due to entrapment and in down gaze due to a reverse leash effect. Identifying all of the positions in which a limitation exists is important to a successful surgical strategy.

Forced Duction Test. A forced duction test is performed by grasping the muscle insertion 90° away from the muscle being evaluated (Fig. 6–1). In the case of the inferior rectus, the insertions of the medial and lateral rectus muscles are grasped with toothed forceps, and the eye is gently elevated and depressed. Care must be exercised not to retropulse the globe, as this may give a false-negative result.

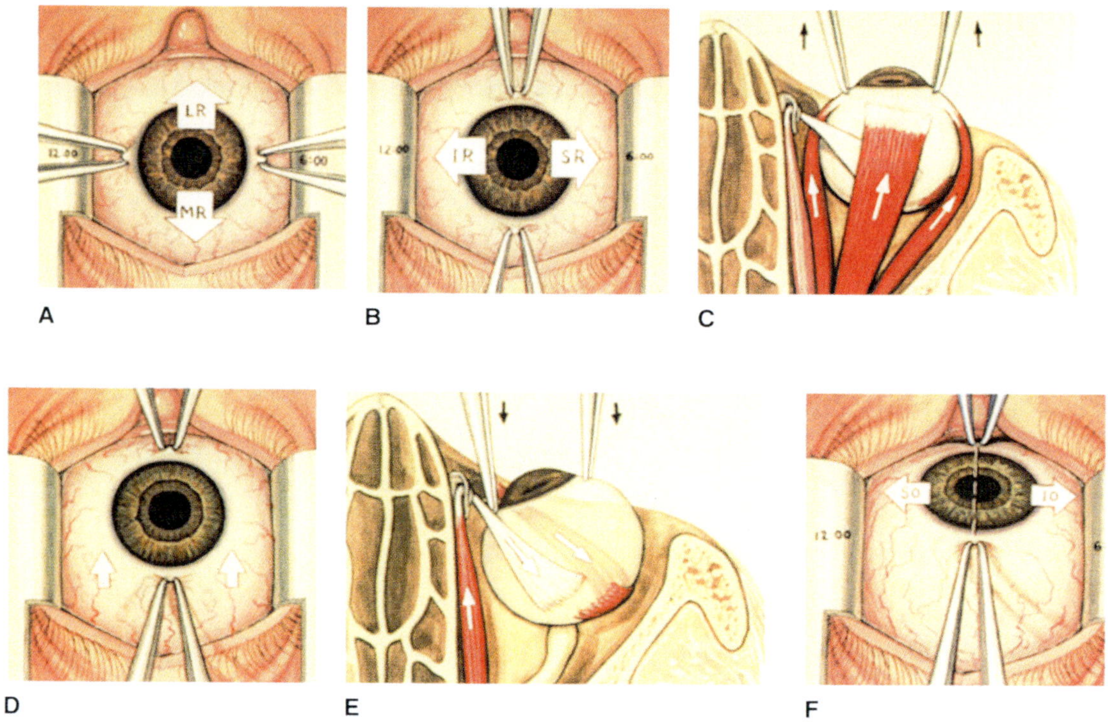

Figure 6–1. Classical forced duction test. For a rectus muscle to be placed on stretch, the eye must be lifted anteriorly out of the orbit. The conjunctiva and sclera are grasped 2.0 mm posterior to the limbus with toothed forceps, which are placed opposite each other 90° from the muscle being tested. The forceps are lifted gently, mildly proptosing the eye from the orbit. This allows for easy determination of any restriction or limitation of movement. (*A*) To test horizontal rectus muscles, the limbus is grasped at the 12 and 6 o'clock positions and the eye is lifted gently. The eye is rotated nasally to test the lateral rectus and laterally to test the medial rectus. The eye should move freely in either direction. If restriction is encountered (positive force duction), the eye is retropulsed to see if restriction improves. If it does not, then it may be caused by a nonrectus abnormality, such as periocular scarring or other orbital cause. (*B*) To test vertical rectus muscles, the limbus is grasped at the 3 and 9 o'clock positions. The eye is gently elevated and rotated inferiorly to test the superior rectus and superiorly to test the inferior rectus. If restriction is encountered, it can be further evaluated as outlined in part A. (*C*) For the rectus muscle to be placed on stretch, the eye must be lifted anteriorly out of the orbit. The conjunctiva and sclera are grasped 2.0 mm posterior to the limbus with toothed forceps, which are placed opposite each other 90° from the muscle being tested. The forceps are lifted gently, mildly proptosing the eye from the orbit. This allows for easy determination of any restriction or limitation of movement. (*D,E*) To evaluate oblique muscles, the limbus is grasped with toothed forceps at the 3 and 9 o'clock positions. The eye should be rotated nasally and retropulsed. By retropulsion of the eye in the adducted position, the superior and inferior oblique muscles are placed on maximum stretch. (*F*) Moving the eye upward tests the superior oblique, and moving the eye downward tests the inferior oblique. While this test is performed, the most important forceps are located nasally over the medial rectus muscle insertion. It is in the nasal forceps that the examiner will first sense restriction. As the eye is elevated or depressed, the nasal forceps will become limited and the eye will begin to twist or tort. This feeling is different than the one that occurs when testing rectus muscles, in which restriction is felt equally in both forceps. It is important to keep the imaginary line between the forceps parallel to the floor of the orbit while moving the eye superiorly and inferiorly in adduction.

Retropulsion, however, can be used to confirm the suspicion that a rectus muscle restriction exists, since this maneuver will lessen the muscle tightness and improve the duction. Just the opposite occurs from restriction caused by either oblique muscle. Because the oblique muscle insertions attach posterior to their effective origins, retropulsion actually tightens the muscle rather than loosening it. Thus, when forced duction tests are performed on these muscles, they should be retropulsed and then elevated or depressed (see Chapter 3, "Oblique Muscle Dysfunction").

The object of any forced duction test is to compare the amount of movement the examiner can achieve with the amount that the patient was able to achieve. This is important, as often there is a paralytic component to the strabismus.

Forced Generation Test. A useful adjunct test is the force generation assessment. In restrictive situations, it can be difficult to determine whether there is a paretic component just by observing ocular rotations. The force generation test can be useful in these situations. The test is performed by having the patient look away from the field of action of the muscle being tested. After application of topical anesthesia, the muscle insertion is grasped with toothed forceps and the patient is asked to look slowly in the direction of the muscle's primary field of action. A subjective evaluation is then made by resisting the rotation. If uncertainty exists as to the amount of power generated by the muscle, the same muscle on the other eye can be similarly evaluated.

Caution must be exercised to avoid tearing the conjunctiva or scratching the cornea. The key maneuver to avoid these complications is to have the patient look *slowly* and to have a firm grasp of the tissue. In older individuals, it is almost impossible not to cause a small subconjunctival hemorrhage with this test. It is important to warn the patient that this will occur. Grasping the muscle insertion rather than the limbal area will minimize this problem.

Inspection of Surrounding Tissue. Careful inspection of the surrounding tissue is necessary to identify any factors contributing to the ocular rotation defect. Conjunctival scarring, previous orbital or eye surgery, or bony orbital changes can affect eye movement. Conjunctival scarring can limit ocular rotation in two ways:

1. A fibrotic band of conjunctival tissue can act as a leash, holding the eye and preventing movement.
2. Conversely, fibrotic conjunctiva can also prevent movement by not relaxing (reverse leash). Thus, the restrictive abnormality may actually be on the opposite side.

For example, an eye may not be able to abduct because of conjunctival scarring over the lateral rectus, as opposed to medial rectus restriction. Observing the behavior of the eye as it moves into lateral gaze is helpful in distinguishing between these two entities. With medial rectus restriction, the eye usually retracts into the orbit on attempted abduction. With lateral conjunctival scarring there is no retraction of the globe, but rather retraction of the conjunctival tissue overlying the lateral rectus.

Previous orbital or ocular surgery can have a dramatic effect on the tissue surrounding the globe. This is especially true in patients who have had orbital exploration for trauma, orbital decompression for thyroid ophthalmopathy, repair of blowout fractures with implants, or scleral buckling procedures. Extensive manipulation of Tenon's tissue and orbital fat can result in significant scarring and fibrotic changes that limit normal ocular rotation. A thorough review of previous surgical procedures can be helpful in understanding the cause of the current motility disturbance.

For example, in a patient with a vertical muscle imbalance after retinal detachment surgery, knowledge of the location and size of the exoplant is important when preparing the strabismus surgical plan. It may be that a large superior exoplant is limiting movement of the eye and must be removed. Conversely, extensive manipulation and cryo treatment inferiorly may be causing a restriction to elevation.

Eyes that are enophthalmic, proptotic, or otherwise displaced may respond unpredictably to strabismus surgery. The displacement of normal structures causes the force vectors to be altered, along with muscle pulleys and other supporting tissues. This shift may enhance or limit the effectiveness of muscle recession and resection procedures. Enophthalmos and proptosis signal changes in the surrounding fat and connective tissue that may contribute to abnormal ocular movement. For example, in patients with thyroid myopathy, the entire orbital contents may be altered and restriction to movement may be due to fibrotic changes in tissue other than the extraocular muscles.

SURGICAL CONCEPTS

Relieving the Restriction. The overriding principle in treating restrictive strabismus is to relieve the restriction. The more limited the movement, the more this becomes necessary. Improving the restrictive component is generally accomplished with muscle-loosening/weakening procedures such as recessions. Unfortunately, this creates a problem that is manifested by reduced rotation in the field of action of the weakened muscle. Thus, while simply recessing the involved muscles will improve the strabismus, the optimal result cannot be obtained without addressing the iatrogenic strabismus that results. *The most successful surgical strategy is one that maximally improves the motility defect while minimally inducing new strabismus in other gaze positions.* This usually requires surgery on multiple muscles involving both eyes.

Creating a Matching Limitation. In some circumstances, it is necessary to create a matching limitation of movement in the normal eye. In all restrictive conditions, in addition to limitation of movement in one eye, there is an associated overaction of the antagonist to the yoke muscle in the other eye. For example, in a left medial wall blowout fracture, the left eye will not rotate outward; therefore, there is a resultant overaction of the left lateral rectus muscle's yoke muscle (the right medial rectus). A weakening procedure (recession or fadenoperation) on the right medial rectus muscle can facilitate realignment of the eyes.

In some circumstances, if the restriction is mild and due to extensive scarring or previous orbital trauma, it may be advisable to avoid manipulation of the involved eye altogether. In this case, a weakening procedure of the contralateral antagonist muscle alone can give a satisfactory result. For example, in a patient with a left medial wall blowout fracture with a residual esotropia on left lateral gaze due to left medial rectus restriction, a recession of the contralateral right medial rectus can eliminate the strabismus while avoiding surgery on the already compromised left medial rectus. In this case, matching the weakness in the normal right eye to the limitation in the involved left eye gives a predictable outcome and avoids the need to manipulate the already damaged tissue.

COMMENT

Gunter K. von Noorden, MD

Treating a limitation of ocular motility by creating a matching limitation of the yoke muscle in the fellow eye is a valid option in certain forms of paralytic or restrictive strabismus. The effect and consequences of this procedure must be clearly understood. This operation will produce a conjugate gaze paresis. I have often heard and read that this artificial paresis will enlarge the field of single binocular vision. This is not the case, but the frequency of a patient's awareness of diplopia will be decreased in the paretic gaze position when the secondary overaction of the yoke muscle is dampened by a recession or retroequatorial myopexy.

Combined Restriction and Paresis. Many of the motility disturbances that are classified as restrictive are really a combination of restriction and paresis. Such entities as thyroid myopathy, blowout fractures, and postcataract strabismus have a paralytic component to the disorder. This may be due to nerve injury or altered muscle dynamics that mimic paresis. Regardless of the cause, the behavior is similar. This creates a dilemma for the strabismus surgeon. To treat the restriction, the surgeon normally recesses or weakens the muscle. This approach, however, results in an exaggerated underaction if the muscle's function was also compromised. In this situation, if the restriction must be relieved, then an additional procedure should be performed to weaken the yoke muscle on the other eye.

For example, a patient with thyroid myopathy has a tight inferior rectus and is fusing in down gaze. A recession of this muscle will improve the vertical deviation in the primary position but will create diplopia in down gaze because the inferior rectus, which was already compromised by fibrous infiltration, was weakened. Treatment of the induced down-gaze diplopia will require either a small recession or a fadenoperation of the contralateral inferior rectus.

In some circumstances, excessive weakening of the restricted muscle, necessary to obtain primary-position alignment, can be avoided by simultaneously weakening the overacting muscle on the normal eye (that is, matching the limitation). In the previous example, this would mean performing a recession on the contralateral superior rectus in combination with, or instead of, weakening the ipsilateral inferior rectus. This has the benefit of retaining as much function as possible of the already compromised muscle while addressing the strabismus that the restriction is creating. Anticipating the possible deleterious effect on ocular rotations of the proposed surgical plan is a helpful exercise that allows for an adjustment in the surgical strategy.

SURGICAL TECHNIQUES

Muscle-weakening procedures are generally necessary to treat restrictive strabismus. These include muscle recession, fadenoperation, myectomy, myotomy, and tenotomy (spacer). Whenever possible, use of the adjustable suture technique is advisable, as the results when using standard surgery amounts can be unpredictable due to altered muscle dynamics, the condition of the surrounding tissue, and the presence of both restriction and paresis. As a general rule, rectus recessions should be conservative. This is true whether they are performed with or without adjustable sutures. When using adjustable sutures the concept that it is easier to advance than to further recess does not apply to tight, restricted muscles. In general, large recessions tend to create unwanted new deviations, necessitating additional surgery.

COMMENT

Marshall M. Parks, MD

The logic the author uses in devising his surgical plans to manage the various causes of restriction is unassailable. However, the technique developed and employed to execute the surgical plan is individual for each surgeon: It becomes her or his surgical signature. My signature is different from Dr Buckley's. His incorporates a large portion of the adjustable suture technique, which, of course, requires the hangback of the muscle rather than the fixed suture attaching the muscle to the globe, permitting changing the scleral site to which the muscle reattaches as determined by a postoperative examination and adjustment. Philosophies vary among surgeons as to which technique is more beneficial to the final outcome measured 6 weeks or more postoperatively. So far as I am aware, neither technique can claim to reduce the need for reoperation, which, by the way, is so prevalent in managing strabismus that includes restriction of motility in one or both eyes. Therefore, every surgeon should give thought to the question "What in my surgical technique would provide the least distorted or scarred tissue to be contended with at reoperation?"

Hangback recessions are effective and can be used in most situations. There has been some concern about their use on inferior rectus muscles that are tight and require large recessions. In this circumstance, suturing the muscle to the globe may help avoid late overcorrections.

THYROID OPHTHALMOPATHY

Thyroid ophthalmopathy is generally believed to be an autoimmune disorder, characterized by congestion and inflammation of the orbit and surrounding tissues. Clinically, it is most commonly associated with Graves' disease, which consists of hyperthyroidism, infiltrative orbitopathy, and infiltrative dermopathy. Orbital involvement in Graves' disease may appear prior to, or concomitant with, systemic signs of thyroid dysfunction or may appear only after the thyrotoxic state is controlled.

The ocular myopathy does not necessarily reflect the state of thyroid activity. A systemic evaluation may reveal hyperthyroidism, euthyroidism, or even hypothyroidism. The disease can even occur in patients with previously undiagnosed episodes of hyperthyroidism and in those who have had a thyroidectomy. Control of the thyroid condition has little or no effect on the ophthalmic condition. Some evidence indicates that thyroid ablation with radioactive iodine may actually increase the risk of eye abnormalities.

The exact cause of thyroid ophthalmopathy is unknown. There is no doubt that it is in some way connected to thyroid dysfunction, but the exact mechanism is uncertain. Current research has implicated an immunologic response as the underlying cause of the thyroid disease. It is likely that the orbital disease is caused by a similar mechanism, with the target organs being the retro-orbital fat, extraocular muscles, and lacrimal glands. It is interesting that about 5% of patients with Graves' disease also develop myasthenia gravis. Both conditions are mediated by autoantibodies to membrane receptors.

Ocular Findings. The initial symptoms of thyroid ophthalmopathy are usually the result of orbital soft tissue congestion. Conjunctival injection and erythema are typically seen over the horizontal rectus insertions. The conjunctiva is often chemotic, and symptoms of exposure and dry eyes are common. Eyelid retraction is often associated with lid lag. Periorbital edema occurs as the extraocular muscles become swollen. Eventually, proptosis occurs.

The onset of diplopia usually begins slowly and is closely related to the development of exophthalmos. As the extraocular muscles swell, the ocular rotations become limited. The most frequently affected muscle in thyroid disease is the inferior rectus, followed by the medial rectus. Early in the process, patients develop a head position to control diplopia. This is usually a chin-up posture due to a tight inferior rectus, or if the medial rectus is more involved, a head turn to the right or left may be adopted. As the process continues, all the extraocular muscles may become infiltrated, resulting in bizarre motility patterns. During this acute inflammatory phase, there may be pain or a pulling sensation on attempted ocular movement. This usually subsides when the condition moves into the chronic fibrotic stage.

The course of the extraocular muscle involvement varies among patients. Some have a motility disturbance that lasts anywhere from 3 to 12 months and then slowly resolves. However, the patient may be left with persistent orbital congestion, proptosis, or lid retraction. It is possible, although rare, to have no permanent residual ocular abnormalities. If the disorder progresses to the fibrotic stage, persistent diplopia often results. Surgical intervention can be considered if the disease course and motility measurements have been stable for at least 4 to 6 months. It is also important to ensure that thyroid function has been adequately controlled and is stable. If thyroid ablation or removal is contemplated, eye surgery should be delayed until this has been completed.

Diagnosis. The diagnosis of thyroid ophthalmopathy can be made by clinical examination, laboratory testing, and orbital computed tomography (CT) or magnetic resonance imaging (MRI) scans (Fig. 6–2). The typical presentation of proptosis, acquired vertical diplopia, and lid retraction is present in the majority of patients.

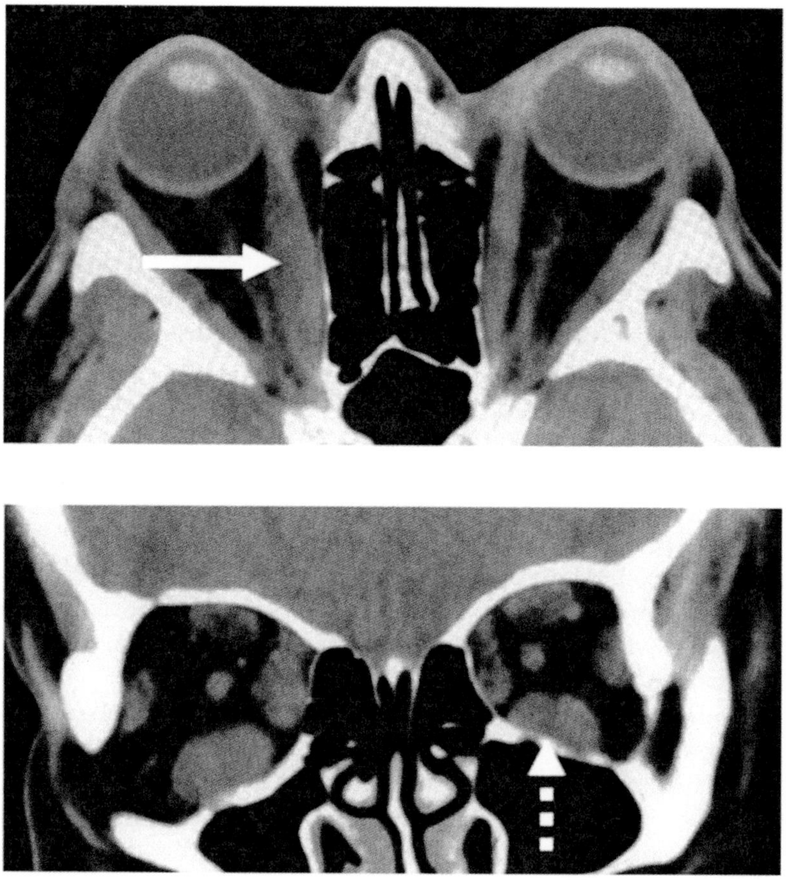

A

B

Figure 6–2. Thyroid myopathy. (*A*) Axial computed tomography (CT) scan showing enlargement of the medial rectus muscles. Note that enlargement occurs posterior to the globe (*white arrow*). Optic nerve compromise can occur if enlargement extends to the orbital apex. (*B*) Coronal CT scan showing enlargement of the inferior rectus muscles (*dashed arrow*). While the inferior and medial rectus muscles are most commonly involved, all muscles usually have some enlargement.

The ocular evaluation should include measurement of exophthalmos, assessment of ocular rotations including motility measurements, forced duction and force generation determination, and visual field measurement. Not infrequently, patients with thyroid ophthalmopathy have normal thyroid function studies at T_3 (triiodothyronine) and T_4 (thyroxine), but thyroid-stimulating hormone (TSH, thyrotropin)) is often reduced.

The CT findings are very characteristic, showing enlargement of one or more of the extraocular muscles with proptosis. Muscle involvement is almost always bilateral, with the muscle enlargement usually involving the muscle belly and sparing the tendon. If the clinical presentation is typical for thyroid ophthalmopathy and no evidence of optic nerve compromise is present, CT or MRI scans are not needed. If the diagnosis is in question, an unenhanced orbital CT scan is recommended.

Surgical Treatment. The general principles of strabismus surgery are outlined in Table 6–1. Once the acute orbital inflammatory phase has resolved, persistent diplopia can be addressed surgically. If orbital surgery is necessary, it should be performed before strabismus surgery (Fig. 6–3). The waiting time varies among individuals, but a minimum of 4 to 6 months of stable strabismus measurements and ocular rotations is reasonable before suggesting muscle surgery. At this stage, the muscle dynamics have been altered, with normal elasticity and contractility becoming significantly impaired. These changes affect the response to surgical manipulation and contribute to the unpredictable postoperative results that are often seen.

The muscles most commonly involved are the inferior rectus and medial rectus. The disease process is usually asymmetric, and often both vertical and horizontal problems coexist. Since the muscles involved are large and fibrotic, recession procedures are preferred. Adjustable sutures can be very helpful, since the normal muscle dose–response curves are difficult to generalize to this patient population. If adjustable sutures are used, postoperative goals should aim for a slight under-

Table 6–1 Surgical Principles for Thyroid Motility Disorders

1. Deviation should be stable for 4 to 6 months.
2. Thyroid dysfunction should be properly controlled medically.
3. If orbital decompression is contemplated, motility surgery should be delayed until after orbital surgery.
4. Lid position is often altered following motility surgery.
5. Recessions are used whenever possible. (Resecting a fibrotic muscle will result in restriction of movement.)
6. Adjustable sutures are used in severe restrictions. (Surgeon should beware of overcorrecting, aiming for slight undercorrection at adjustment.)
7. Surgeon should aim for single binocular vision in primary and down-gaze positions.
8. For complicated vertical and horizontal deviations, operations should be staged.
9. Extreme care should be exercised in handling the conjunctiva, which is usually thin and tears easily.
10. Postoperative exposure can be a serious problem, especially in large inferior rectus recessions.
11. Ocular tissue ischemia can occur in the conjunctiva, sclera, and anterior segment.

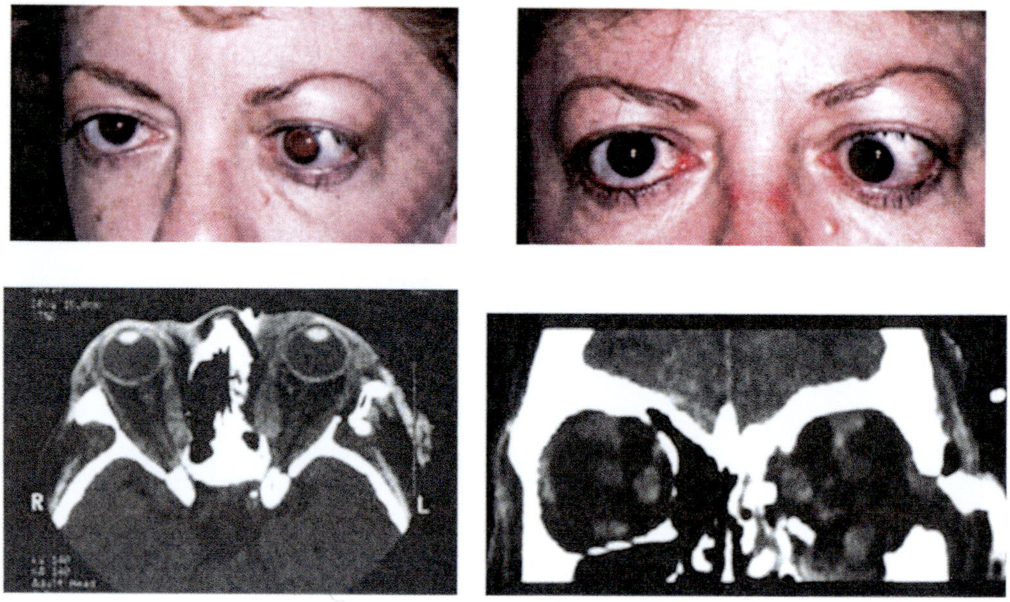

A B

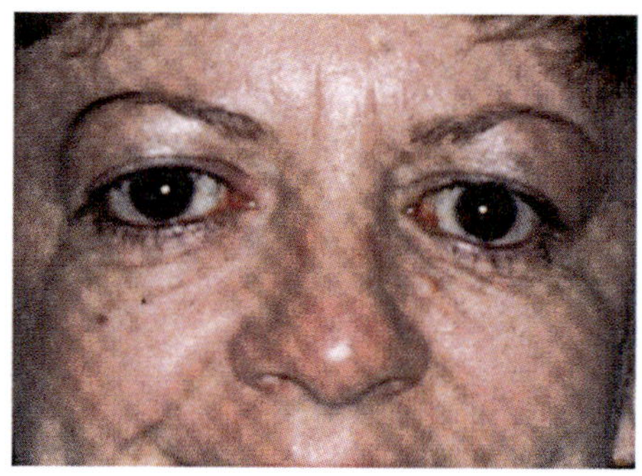

C

Figure 6–3. Orbital decompression. (*A*) Patient with significant thyroid myopathy, with marked proptosis and limitation of movement of the left eye. A computed tomography scan shows enlargement of the medial and inferior rectus muscles. (*B*) Orbital decompression was performed on the left eye, with the floor and medial and lateral walls removed. Note the marked reduction in the amount of proptosis but no real change in ocular motility. (*C*) The patient after recession of both medial rectus muscles and the left inferior rectus.

correction for both esotropia and hypotropia, as there typically is a late drift toward overcorrection. This is especially true for inferior rectus recessions, which are notorious for this phenomenon.

COMMENT

Gunter K. von Noorden, MD

Concerning the use of adjustable sutures during inferior rectus recession in endocrine myopathy, I was in favor of it until I had two patients in whom these sutures became untied and the muscle slipped 3 and 10 days after surgery, respectively. Needless to say, after this experience, I no longer advocate the use of adjustable sutures in this condition. This outcome has been reported by others as well.

Since complete restoration of binocular function in all gaze positions is rarely achieved, priority should be given to eliminating diplopia in primary gaze and down gaze. The more horizontal movement that can be made before diplopia occurs, the more functional the patient will be. A very narrow window is difficult to use while walking, driving, and performing tasks in which the head or body is moving. When compromises must be made, a wider area of single vision is preferable to a centered one, provided that a large, abnormal head posture is not required.

Patients with thyroid ophthalmopathy tend to be older and therefore have thin conjunctiva, with sparse anterior Tenon's tissue. This, coupled with proptosis, often makes closure of the conjunctiva difficult. *Extra care must be exercised to preserve as much of this tissue as possible.* Avoidance of excessive manipulation, stretching, and traction on this tissue is advisable. Limbal incisions are generally preferred over fornix incisions for this reason. Reoperations are also made more difficult if the conjunctiva has been handled poorly during the primary operation.

Surgical approach. The surgical approach to correcting strabismus in thyroid ophthalmopathy depends on whether the patient has an esotropia, a hypertropia or hypotropia, late overcorrection after previous strabismus surgery, or A-pattern strabismus.

1. *Esotropia:* Patients with an esotropia due to thyroid myopathy respond well to medial rectus recession surgery. In most circumstances, both eyes are involved and therefore both medial rectus muscles should be recessed (Fig. 6–4). Since these muscles are generally stiff and inelastic, the initial 2.0 to 4.0 mm of recession has a minimal effect on the amount of esotropia. As the recession gets larger, each additional millimeter results in an increasingly large horizontal correction. *Therefore, larger than normal recessions are usually necessary for small deviations*, and *smaller than normal recessions are advisable for large deviations.*

   There is also a tendency for late drift toward exodeviation with time. Whether this is due to medial rectus dynamics, concomitant lateral rectus involvement, or both is unknown. Thus, when the recession is performed using the adjustable suture technique, the ideal postadjustment deviation should be on the esotropic side, just enough to allow fusion, but with as much esophoria as possible. This esodeviation will decrease as the tissues heal.

   Lateral rectus resections can be used to treat residual esodeviations after the medial rectus muscle has been recessed, but primary resections are not very effective and should be avoided. Forced duction testing is important in assessing how much residual restriction remains and is helpful in selecting the appropriate second procedure for a residual esotropia. If the rotation is still significantly limited, then further medial rectus recession may be necessary. As indicated above, further recession amounts should be small to avoid overcorrection. If the deviation is small and the rotation is only mildly involved, then lateral rectus surgery can be performed.

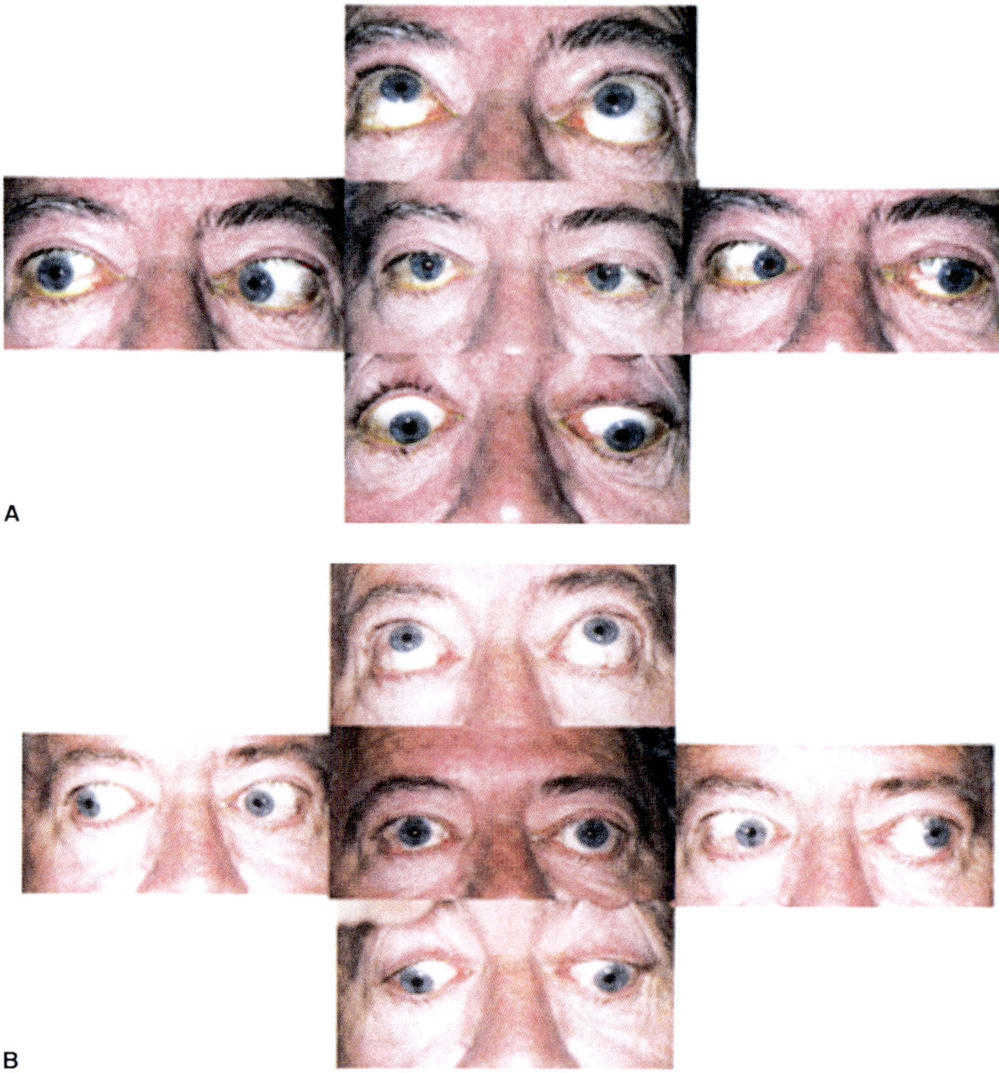

A

B

Figure 6–4. Esotropia secondary to bilateral thyroid eye disease. (*A*) Note the limitation of abduction bilaterally and the mild A pattern, with eyes straight on down gaze. (*B*) The patient after medial rectus recessions. Note the good alignment in the primary position, with improved lateral gaze. The patient has a persistent A pattern, with exotropia on down gaze. This can be improved by supraplacing the medial rectus muscles at the time of recession. Superior oblique posterior tenotomies can also be used.

COMMENT

M. Edward Wilson, MD

When treating esotropia from thyroid myopathy, an important caveat about the dose–response curve (mentioned by the author) needs emphasis. Larger than expected recessions are needed for smaller deviations, yet smaller than expected recessions will correct large deviations.

Table 6–2 Surgical Option, Hypotropia, for Thyroid Motility Disorders

Up-gaze deviation	40Δ	30Δ	35Δ	35Δ
Primary deviation	20Δ	20Δ	25Δ	30Δ
Down-gaze deviation	0Δ	10Δ	15Δ	25Δ
Involved eye	Recession IR	Recession IR	Recession IR	Recession IR
Contralateral eye	Fadenoperation IR	Recession SR or (asymmetric recession IR)	Recession SR	

IR = inferior rectus; SR = superior rectus.

2. *Hypertropia or hypotropia:* The most common cause of a vertical deviation is inferior rectus restriction. This is often bilateral but asymmetric. The surgical treatment selected depends on the degree of restriction and the amount of vertical deviation present in down gaze (Table 6–2). As with medial rectus surgery, late overcorrections are common after inferior rectus recessions, so these need to be conservative.

   A common presentation is for the patient to have a hypotropia with no vertical deviation on down gaze, allowing the use of a head position (chin up) to take advantage of this area of single vision. Forced duction testing shows a tight, restricted inferior rectus; clinically, the deviation becomes more pronounced as the patient attempts to look up.

   Surgical weakening of the restricted inferior rectus is required, but this will create a hypertropia postoperatively on down gaze. This inevitable outcome must be addressed by bilateral inferior rectus surgery, either bilateral asymmetric recessions or unilateral recession with a contralateral fadenoperation that can be performed at the same time or as a subsequent procedure (Fig. 6–5). To minimize the size of the resultant hypertropia on down gaze, a recession just large enough to allow comfortable single vision in the pri-

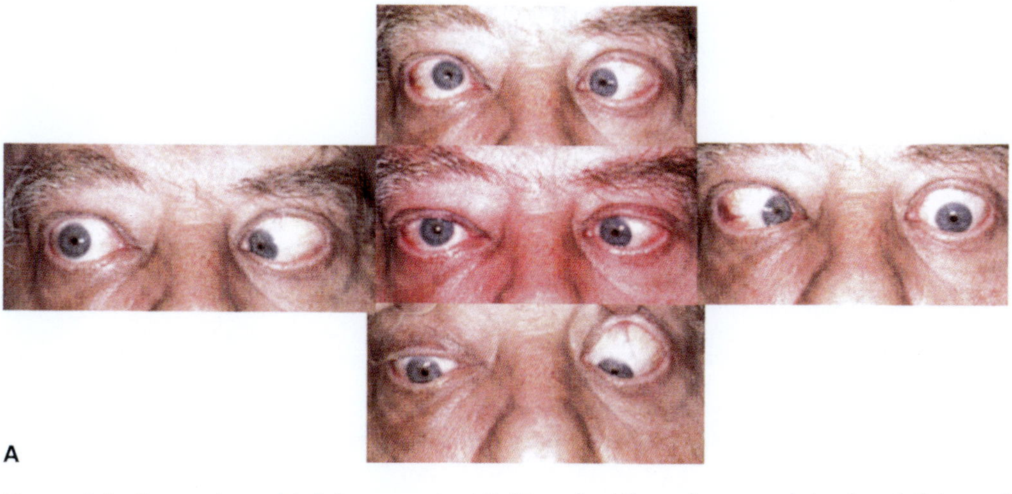

A

Figure 6–5. Esotropia and left hypotropia. (*A*) Note the bilateral severe abduction deficits and bilateral inability to elevate both eyes.

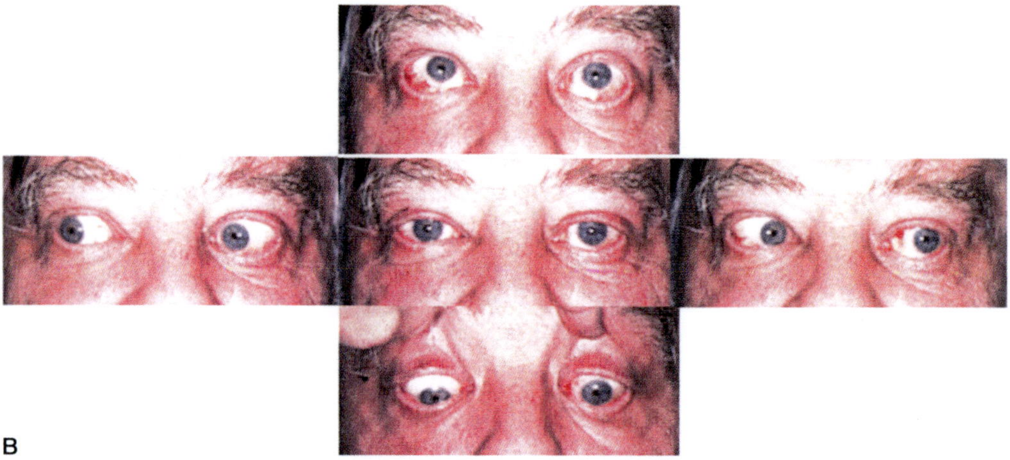

B

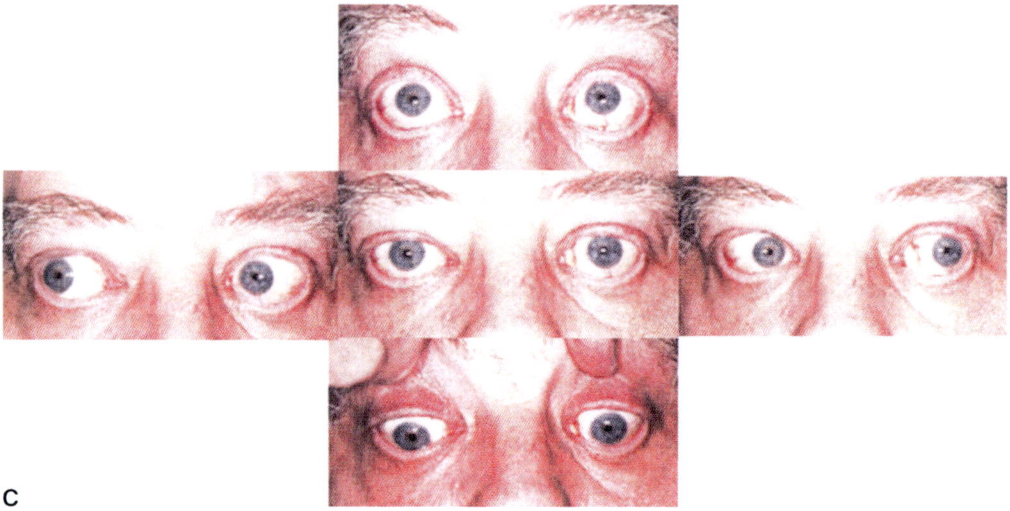

C

Figure 6–5. Esotropia and left hypotropia. (*B*) The patient after bilateral medial rectus recessions and left inferior rectus recessions. Note the improved horizontal motility and single vision in the primary position; however, the patient now has left hypertropia on down gaze. (*C*) The patient after right inferior and medial rectus fadenoperation. Note the marked improvement on down gaze. Combining unilateral recession with contralateral fadenoperation or performing asymmetric bilateral inferior rectus recessions is usually necessary if the patient has bilateral disease.

mary position is advisable. Attempts to achieve normal elevation of the eye will usually weaken the downward rotation excessively, making the resultant down-gaze diplopia more difficult to treat. When adjustable sutures are used, a small residual hypotropia should be present at the end of the adjustment. This will normally improve in 2 to 4 weeks.

The larger the deviation on down gaze, the more likely it can be treated with a single muscle recession or a combination of ipsilateral inferior rectus recession and contralateral superior rectus recession (see Table 6–2). The latter approach helps to decrease the amount of inferior rectus recession necessary to eliminate diplopia in primary gaze, thereby preserving the down-gaze function of the muscle. The ipsilateral inferior rectus is recessed until the down-gaze deviation is corrected, and then the contralateral superior rectus is recessed for the residual vertical deviation in primary gaze. Care must be exercised with this approach if the inferior rectus on the contralateral side is also tight. In this circumstance, recession of the contralateral superior rectus will result in further contracture and restriction of the contralateral inferior rectus, with a resultant large contralateral hypotropia postoperatively. A safer approach is to perform asymmetric inferior rectus recessions or to be very conservative in the amount of superior rectus recession.

3. *Late overcorrection:* The altered muscle dynamics and the presence of asymmetric muscle involvement in patients with thyroid ophthalmopathy make these patients susceptible to late overcorrection after strabismus surgery. This is true for both horizontal and vertical muscle procedures. Judicious dissection of surrounding muscle attachments, use of nonabsorbable sutures, and avoidance of adjustable sutures (and hangback recession without adjustment) have all been advocated to reduce this possibility. The cause of overcorrection is most likely multifactorial, and no single adjustment to surgical technique will eliminate this problem. As a general rule, performing surgery that aims for a slight undercorrection can minimize this risk.
4. *A-pattern strabismus:* The treatment of strabismus in thyroid ophthalmopathy usually involves weakening one or more inferior or medial rectus muscles. This often results in an A-pattern strabismus postoperatively, especially when rectus muscles in both eyes are recessed (Fig. 6–6; see also Figure 6–4). Making an adjustment when reattaching these muscles in anticipation that an A pattern will occur can lessen the impact. Therefore, when both medial rectus muscles are recessed, they should be supraplaced and both inferior

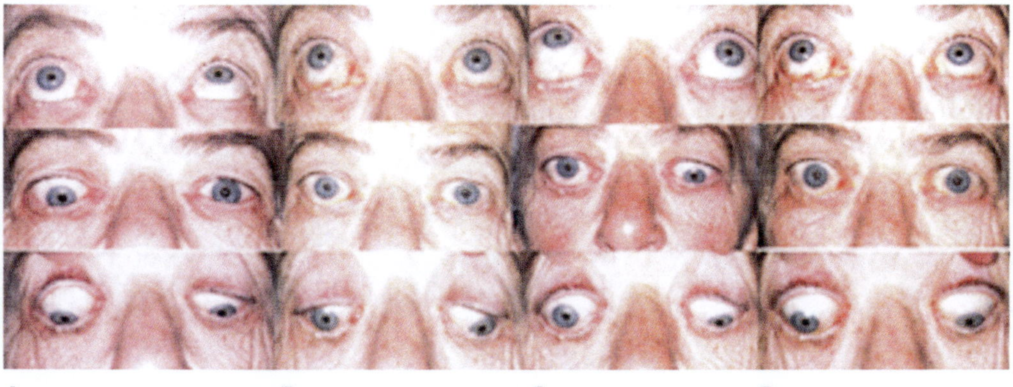

Figure 6–6. Late overcorrection of the A pattern. (*A*) A patient with right hypotropia and a tight right inferior rectus. The patient could fuse in extreme down gaze. (*B*) The patient after right inferior and left superior rectus recession. Note the good alignment in the primary position but right hypertropia on down gaze with the A pattern. (C) About 4 weeks later, the patient developed severe left hypotropia, with decreased elevation of the left eye. Forced duction testing showed significant restriction of elevation of the left eye, indicating a tight left inferior rectus. (D) The patient after left inferior rectus recession, with nasal displacement for the A pattern. Primary alignment has been restored and ocular motility is essentially normal, except for down gaze, where small right hypertropia persists. The patient was able to read without difficulty.

rectus muscles should be medially displaced. This will reduce, but not completely eliminate, the problem.

An alternative approach involves bilateral superior oblique weakening, with either recession, posterior tenotomy, spacer, or nasal tenectomy. The degree of aggressiveness used to weaken the superior oblique in a fusing adult must be carefully titrated. Torsional problems that can occur after bilateral superior oblique weakening procedures that can be difficult to remedy.

ORBITAL WALL FRACTURES

Orbital wall fractures can occur from a variety of traumatic injuries to the face. Typically, an object such as a ball or fist strikes the orbital rim and causes a sudden rise in the pressure of the orbital contents, resulting in a fracture of the orbital floor (Fig. 6–7) or one or more of the orbital walls. Since the pressure rise occurs inside the orbit, the fractured bone displaces outward, into the adjacent sinus, taking some of the orbital contents as well. In most circumstances, the fracture is hinged like a door, and after the pressure is relieved, the fractured bone swings back toward its previous position, trapping the prolapsed orbital tissue in the process. The term *blowout fracture* has been used to describe this phenomenon.

Clinical Presentation. A wide variety of strabismus patterns can be seen after trauma to the orbit due to a combination of restrictive and paralytic factors. In addition to direct injury to the muscle, orbital bone fractures can affect the surrounding tissues, along with their attachments to adjacent structures. When these restrictive elements are combined with innervational abnormalities, the resultant strabismus can be quite complex.

Typically, a blowout fracture involves the floor of the orbit, with the orbital contents displacing inferiorly into the maxillary sinus (Fig. 6–8). This often results in a hypotropia, with limitation of elevation of the involved eye (Fig. 6–9). The amount of limitation depends on the location of the fracture, the amount of orbital

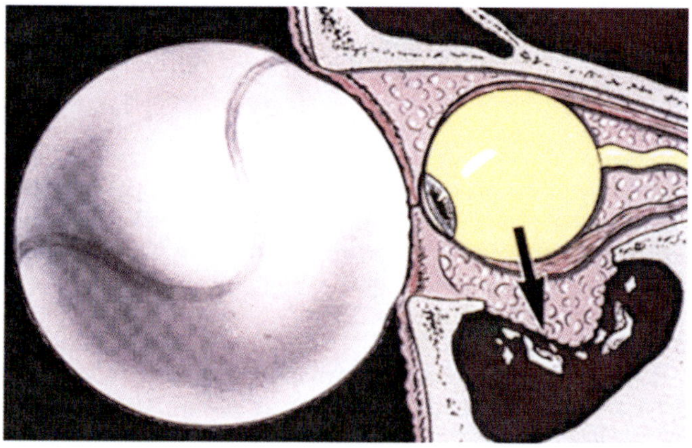

Figure 6–7. Mechanism of orbital floor fracture. An object with a diameter that matches the orbital opening increases orbital pressure, resulting in fracture of the weakest bones.

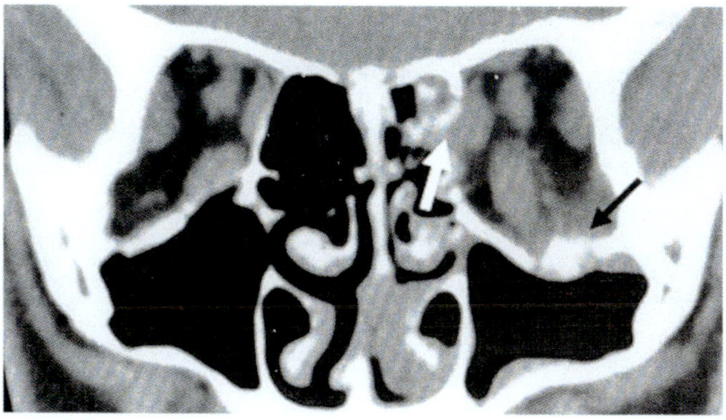

Figure 6–8. Computed tomography scan of the left medial wall and floor fracture. Note the entrapment of the medial rectus in the ethmoid sinus (*white arrow*) and of the inferior rectus in the maxillary sinus (*black arrow*). The patient's motility is shown in Figure 6–10.

tissue trapped in the fracture, and the position of the globe at the moment of impact. Occasionally, a limitation of depression will also occur due to direct injury to the muscle or nerve.

A medial wall fracture can occur in combination with a floor fracture or as an isolated phenomenon. In this circumstance, the medial rectus or its surrounding tissue becomes trapped in the ethmoid bone fracture. This results in an esotropia that worsens on attempted abduction (Fig. 6–10). There may also be a limitation of adduction due to either tethering of the medial rectus (reverse leash) or damage to the muscle or its nerve.

Superior and lateral wall fractures are less common. For strabismus to develop, the fracture usually extends to the orbital rim or involves the zygomatic arch. Fractures in these locations would be expected to cause the same kind of motility disturbance outlined above.

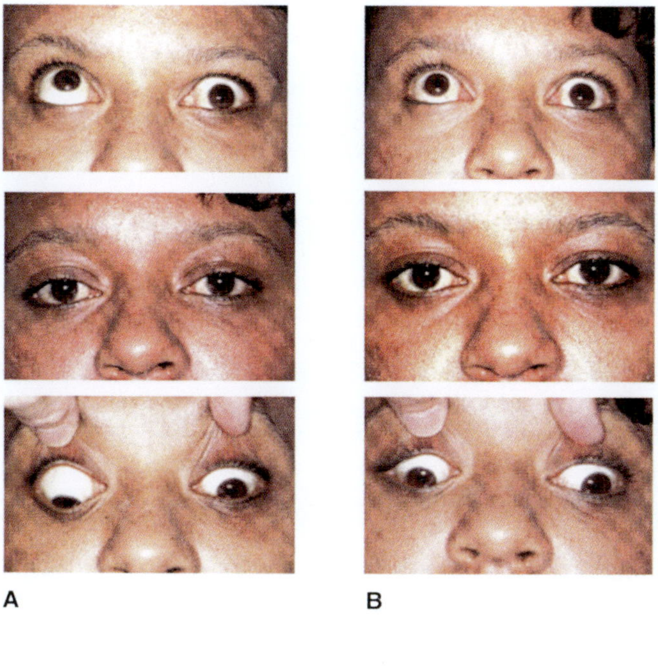

A B

Figure 6–9. Left blowout fracture. (*A*) There is a marked decrease in the elevation and depression of the left eye. Note that the patient is straight in the primary position. (*B*) The patient after recession of the superior and inferior rectus muscles on the right. The patient remains straight in the primary position but is now able to fuse in down gaze. On extreme down gaze, the patient develops small exotropia but can read comfortably.

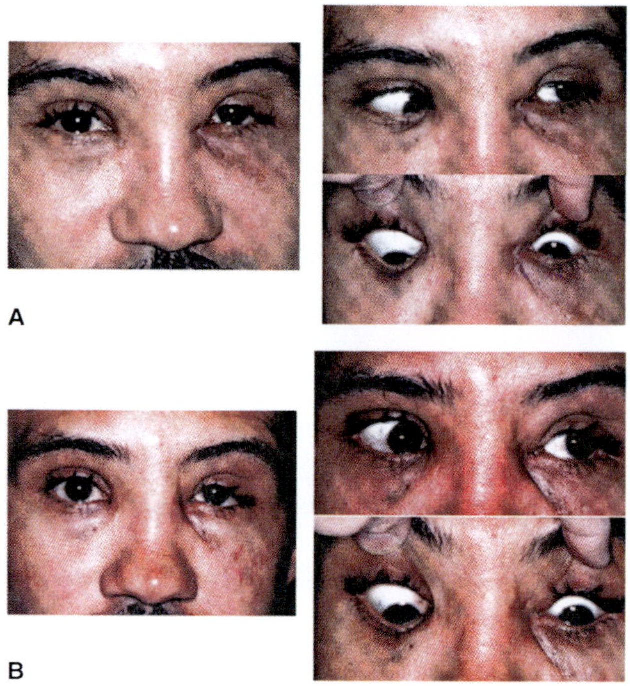

Figure 6–10. Left medial wall and floor fracture. (*A*) The same patient as in Figure 6–8 has no deviation in the primary position, but is limited on down gaze and abduction of the left eye. (*B*) The patient after right medial and inferior rectus fadenoperation. Note the marked improvement in down gaze and lateral-gaze alignment, with preservation of primary gaze.

Diagnosis. The major concern in the evaluation of strabismus secondary to a blowout fracture is whether the motility limitation is due to restriction or paresis. This requires an analysis of forced ductions and force generation. Once the degree of restriction is known, other factors, such as the range of movement, involvement of surrounding tissue, and current areas of single vision, can be incorporated into any surgical plan. Ocular motility measurements, while necessary, are not as important in determining a surgical plan as these other factors.

Particularly important is the range of movement the eye can make before the restriction limits movement. The more limited the rotation, the less likely a simple recession of the involved muscle will be helpful since it will create strabismus in the field of action of that muscle. A typical presentation is for the eye to move relatively normally and then suddenly stop, as if attached to a leash. The *leash effect* represents scarring in and around the muscle. It is always associated with a positive forced duction test.

For example, a patient with a right orbital floor fracture has a limitation of elevation of the right eye. The eye moves normally 20° above midline and then stops. A recession of the right inferior rectus would improve elevation but decrease depression of the right eye. If the range of movement of the involved eye is quite good, then the surgical approach is to create a matching weakness in the other eye by recessing or using the fadenoperation to limit the contralateral antagonist muscle. In the example, this means that a recession or fadenoperation of the left superior rectus would be performed.

The condition of the conjunctival and Tenon's tissues should be evaluated for the presence of scarring or other changes that might limit ocular rotations. If scarring exists, it must be addressed to achieve a satisfactory outcome. In most circumstances, recessing the tight conjunctival tissue will improve ocular rotation.

Neuroimaging. Computed tomography is very helpful in delineating the extent of an orbital fracture and the degree of entrapment of ocular tissues (see Figure 6–8). A nonenhanced thin slice, direct axial, and direct coronal CT scan of the orbits should be performed in all patients with a suspected orbital fracture. Understanding all of the anatomic changes caused by the trauma is necessary to plan the appropriate surgical response. Only patients with strong evidence of muscle or orbital tissue entrapment on CT require orbital surgery for diplopia.

Surgical Treatment.

Timing. The strabismus that results from an orbital fracture can be due to direct muscle injury, entrapment, edema, hemorrhage, or paresis. Distinguishing between these various causes is necessary when planning a surgical approach. The strabismus seen immediately after the trauma is often due to hemorrhage, edema, muscle contusion, or temporary nerve injury and may resolve spontaneously in subsequent weeks. If there is clear CT evidence of extraocular muscle entrapment, orbital surgery should be considered. This is done routinely within the first 2 weeks after injury. Delaying further may result in permanent tissue changes with persistent diplopia.

If the CT scan reveals no enophthalmos or obvious entrapment, orbital surgery for diplopia is not indicated. The diplopia in vast majority of patients in this category, will resolve spontaneously over the next 3 to 4 weeks. Observation is recommended for at least 6 to 8 weeks after trauma or until the edema has resolved. If no improvement has occurred after this time, surgical intervention for strabismus can be considered.

General principles. Patients with strabismus after orbital fractures usually require surgery on both eyes. Patients who have only a restrictive component usually require a recession of the tight muscle. The amount of recession should be kept to the minimum required to achieve alignment in the primary position. Increasing the unrestricted movement further may not be possible without weakening the muscle in its field of action. If weakening the muscle's action cannot be avoided, either a recession or a fadenoperation on the contralateral yoke muscle will be necessary.

In patients with a combined restrictive and paralytic component, this problem is amplified. Under those circumstances, it may be reasonable to avoid surgery on the involved eye altogether and concentrate only on creating a matching weakness in the noninvolved eye.

In many situations, due to either the original orbital trauma or the subsequent orbital surgery, the surrounding tissues are fibrotic and constitute a major component of the restrictive process. Minimizing their impact on ocular rotations is important in achieving a successful surgical outcome. Removing adhesions to the globe and muscles wherever possible is necessary. If it is apparent that fibrous tissue will continue to be a factor postoperatively, holding the eye away from areas of existing fibrous scar formation during the immediate postoperative period is helpful. This prevents these tissues from attaching to the globe anteriorly, thereby decreasing the restrictive effect. Traction sutures or botulinum toxin can be useful for this purpose.

Surgical approach. The types of motility disorders seen after orbital wall fractures can be divided into three main groups: purely restrictive, purely innervational (or paralytic), or a combination of restriction and paresis. Each of these types must be approached differently.

1. *Restriction:* The surgical approach to orbital wall fractures in this category depends on the ocular alignment in the primary-gaze position.
   a. *Primary-gaze deviation:* If there is a deviation in the primary position, a recession of the restricted muscle is necessary. The amount of recession should be limited to what is necessary to correct the deviation in the primary position without causing a significant strabismus in the field of action of the recessed muscle.

      For example, a patient presents after a right orbital floor fracture. There is a right hypotropia in the primary position, with marked limitation of up gaze. A recession of the right inferior rectus can be performed to improve the primary-gaze deviation. Excessive recession of the right inferior rectus will result in a hyperdeviation of the right eye on down gaze and should be avoided if possible. If it cannot be avoided, a fadenoperation on the contralateral left inferior rectus will be necessary to minimize diplopia in down gaze. For vertical deviations, leaving the patient with a residual limitation of up gaze is preferable to creating a hyperdeviation on down gaze.

      With medial wall fractures, residual limitations of rotation become more important. The success of the horizontal surgical procedure is determined by the amount of horizontal movement that can be obtained. Just getting the eye to the primary position is usually unsatisfactory. In this circumstance, surgery on both eyes may be necessary.

      For example, a patient presents with a right medial wall fracture and an esotropia in the primary position, with marked limitation of abduction of the right eye. A recession of the right medial rectus needs to be performed to reduce the restriction of ocular rotations of the right eye. The amount of recession should be enough to enable the right eye to rotate laterally well past midline. Such a recession will undoubtedly result in a weakness of adduction of the right eye, creating an exotropia on left gaze. This will necessitate a recession of the left lateral rectus.
   b. *No primary-gaze deviation:* Some patients have no deviation in the primary position, with an inability to elevate or abduct the eye (see Fig. 6–9). Under these circumstances, surgery of the noninvolved eye will be necessary. In vertical strabismus, recessing the restricted inferior rectus to improve up gaze will undoubtedly create a hyperdeviation in the primary position, as well as in down gaze. If this approach is chosen, a recession and a possible fadenoperation will need to be performed on the con-

tralateral inferior rectus. A potentially more beneficial procedure may be a fadenoperation on the contralateral superior rectus.

In either case, surgery on the noninvolved eye is required. Since very few individuals require diplopia-free up gaze, such patients can be managed conservatively unless occupation or lifestyle requirements necessitate intervention.

As indicated above, the amount of horizontal eye movement is more critical, and single vision in the primary position without much horizontal movement is not optimal. For example, a patient with a right medial wall fracture is orthophoric with a small left head turn but has marked limitation of abduction of the right eye. An attempt to relieve some of the restriction should be made. This can be accomplished by recessing the restricted right medial rectus. Doing so will create an adduction defect, resulting in an exotropia on opposite left lateral gaze. To maintain as wide a field of single binocular vision as possible, a contralateral left lateral rectus recession will be necessary.

2. *Paresis:* If the main component responsible for the strabismus is a paresis of the muscle, the approach outlined in Chapter 5, "Paralytic Strabismus," should be employed. The main factors to be analyzed are residual muscle function and field of greatest deviation. The surgical strategy is to improve paretic muscle function and weaken the contralateral yoke muscles.

   For example, a patient has a right floor fracture, resulting in an inability to fully depress the right eye. Forced duction testing reveals no restriction preventing downward movement of the right eye. Force generation testing indicates that the inferior rectus is weak. The eye can rotate downward about −2. In this situation, the residual muscle function is moderately compromised and the field of greatest deviation is downward in the direction of the involved inferior rectus. The approach advocated in Chapter 5 would be to either resect the right inferior rectus or perform a fadenoperation on the left inferior rectus (Fig. 6–11). If there is a small deviation in the primary position, a recession could be combined with the fadenoperation. For more examples, see Chapter 5.

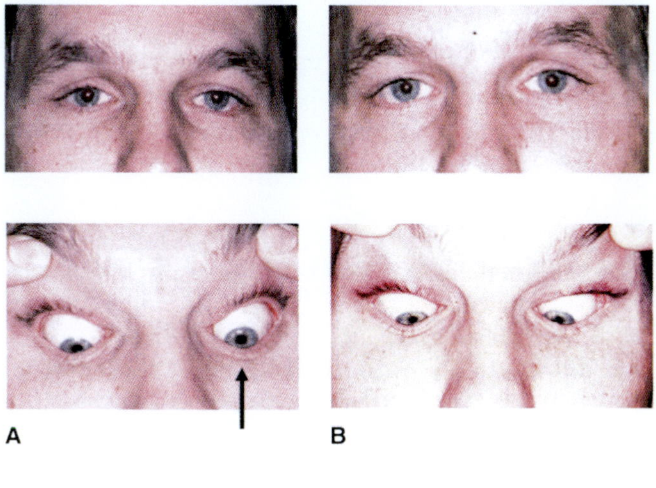

Figure 6–11. Left floor fracture. (*A*) Note the limitation of depression of the left eye (*black arrow*). There is no deviation in the primary position. (*B*) The patient after right inferior rectus fadenoperation. Note the improvement in down-gaze alignment, with retention of primary gaze.

3. *Combined restriction and paresis*
   a. *Primary-gaze deviation:* This is the most difficult situation to treat, since anything that is done to relieve the restriction will make the paresis worse. Therefore, the restrictive component must be dealt with conservatively, recessing the muscle only enough to regain single vision in the primary position. Since relieving the restriction will worsen the paresis, compromises need to be made. In some situations, it will be impossible to preserve much muscle function after the restriction is relaxed, and a transposition procedure may be indicated.

      For example, a patient has a left orbital floor fracture, with a left hypotropia in the primary position and limitation of upward and downward movement. Forced duction testing shows restriction on up gaze but none on down gaze. A recession of the left inferior rectus restores single vision in the primary position but results in a large left hyperdeviation on down gaze. A transposition procedure on the left will be necessary to restore some downward movement of the left eye. This may need to be combined with a fadenoperation on the right inferior rectus.
   b. *No primary-gaze deviation:* If there is no deviation in the primary position, surgery on the uninvolved eye to create a matching weakness is preferred.

      For example, a patient has a left floor fracture, with no deviation in the primary position, but has a limitation on up and down gaze (see Fig. 6–9). Surgery on this eye will not be helpful since improving up gaze will worsen down gaze, and vice versa, unless down gaze is so poor that a transposition procedure is required. Otherwise, creating a matching weakness on the other side is necessary. This can be accomplished through recessions or the fadenoperation.

RETINAL DETACHMENT SURGERY

The incidence of diplopia after retinal detachment surgery has been reported to be as high as 60%. The majority of patients have only transient motility disturbances, which have been attributed to periocular edema, poor vision, or muscle hemorrhage. Recovery is usually rapid, with only 5% of patients experiencing persistent diplopia for more than 3 months.

The causes of the residual strabismus can be divided into four types: mechanical, direct muscle injury, redirection of muscle force vectors, and sensory disruption.

1. *Mechanical causes:* The major cause of mechanical restrictions after retinal surgery is adhesions between extraocular muscles and sclera (especially after diathermy) or fat (fat adherence syndrome). This occurs because Tenon's tissue behind the muscle insertion is violated, resulting in an inflammatory reaction that ultimately causes fibrous changes in the extraconal fat that then attaches to the adjacent periorbital tissue. Attempts to remove these restrictions are frequently unsuccessful because further manipulation of the tissues often rekindles a similar fibrotic response.

COMMENT
Marshall M. Parks, MD

The fat adherence syndrome can be "cured" only by prevention. Most cases result from an improper or careless technique that lacerates Tenon's capsule more than 8.0 mm peripheral to the limbus, allowing the extraconal fat to prolapse into Tenon's space and invariably infiltrate into the sclera and external surface of Tenon's capsule as vascular fibrous tissue restricting the motility of the eye. Also, secondary cicatrization displaces the involved eye's position in the orbit, affecting its alignment with the other eye. Use of artificial membranes, designed to prevent rescarring after extensive freeing of the scleral scarring by sharp dissection, has proven to be futile.

A large or bulky exoplant placed underneath an extraocular muscle effectively shortens the muscle, simulating a resection. If the surrounding tissue becomes fibrotic, limitation of ocular rotation can also occur in the field of action of the involved muscle. Removing the exoplant usually has little effect on the ocular motility abnormality.

2. *Direct muscle injury:* Trauma to the extraocular muscles during retinal surgery can occur from a variety of sources. The most common is excessive stretching, which is often necessary for gaining exposure to apply encircling buckles and exoplants. Some surgeons advocate protective removal of rectus muscles during retinal detachment surgery to minimize damage to the muscles from this prolonged pulling and use of instruments. If a rectus has to be removed to increase exposure during retinal surgery advancement, recession or transposition of the muscle can occur during reattachment. Excessive traction can even result in complete avulsion of a rectus. Muscle rupture after aggressive cryotherapy has also been reported.
3. *Redirection of muscle force vectors:* Exoplants and encircling bands can change the direction of the normal force vectors of the extraocular muscles. The oblique muscles are particularly susceptible to this problem. During placement of an encircling band, the superior oblique tendon can be displaced anteriorly. In this position, the tendon acts like an elevator instead of a depressor, creating a hyperdeviation with incyclotorsion (see Fig. 6–12). Similarly, the inferior oblique can be pulled anteriorly and tucked under a large exoplant, creating a restrictive hypotropia and excyclotorsion.
4. *Sensory disruption:* Loss of fusion can occur after retinal surgery from persistent macular abnormalities or edema, image distortion, induced aniseikonia from silicone oil, aphakia, and anisometropia from elongation by scleral buckling. Macular dysfunction is particularly problematic since many of these patients have peripheral fusion and cannot seem to superimpose the distorted central image on the normal one. This type of diplopia is extremely annoying to the patient and very difficult to remedy. Prolonged periods of poor vision, which sometimes accompany recovery from retinal surgery, can aggravate underlying motility conditions, such as intermittent exotropia or convergence insufficiency. Once the breakdown has occurred, it may persist even if visual function improves.

Diagnosis. Since the majority of retinal breaks causing retinal detachment tend to occur superiorly, vertical deviations are the most common type of strabismus causing diplopia. These deviations can be hypertropia, hypotropia, iatrogenic Brown syndrome, or cyclotropia. Almost all are restrictive in nature, so forced duction testing is crucial in the evaluation.

Horizontal deviations can be divided into two types: comitant deviations, which are usually secondary to visual deprivation, and incomitant deviations, which result from restrictions. Patients with poor visual acuity, macular distortion, and anisometropia secondary to aphakia or silicone oil often develop a sensory esotropia or exotropia. These deviations are almost always comitant and are associated with a negative forced duction test. Careful preoperative evaluation is necessary to determine whether fusion potential exists and to ensure that the patient will not be bothered by intractable double vision if ocular alignment is attempted.

Surgical Treatment. Incomitant horizontal deviations occur infrequently and are most often associated with medial rectus restriction. The intraconal fat pads extend more anteriorly and are easy to violate in this location. Careful clinical evaluation, with forced duction testing, usually identifies the site of restriction. A combination esotropia in one gaze direction, with an associated exodeviation in the opposite direction, indicates a far posterior adhesion.

General principles. Surgical treatment of residual strabismus after retinal detachment surgery may include any or all of the following: removal of the retinal hardware, the adjustable suture technique and hangback recession, surgery on the normal eye, and recession of conjunctiva and Tenon's tissue.

1. *Exoplant and scleral band:* The need to remove the retinal detachment repair hardware to improve ocular motility is controversial. Motility surgery

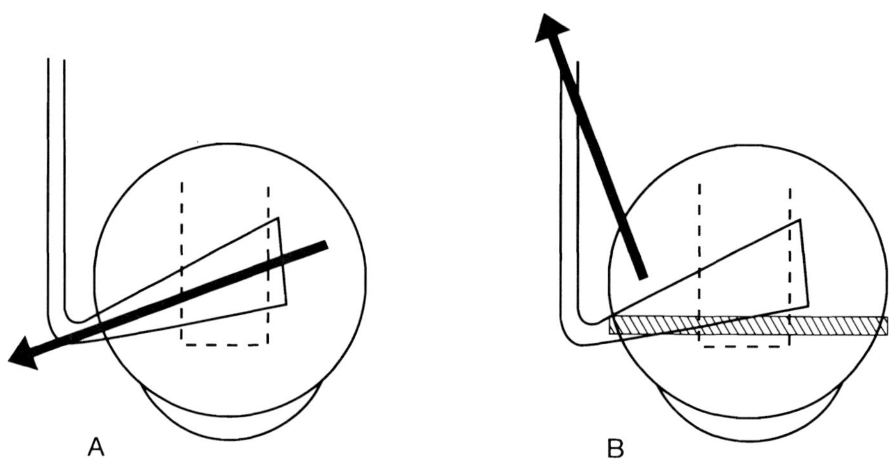

Figure 6–12. Scleral buckle. (*A*) The superior oblique normally depresses, abducts, and intorts the eye. (*B*) When a scleral buckle is placed, the tendon can be trapped, creating new insertion on the anterior nasal side and making the eye elevate, adduct, and extort.

in the presence of a bulky exoplant can be troublesome and is technically difficult. In this situation, removal to gain access to the extraocular muscle seems reasonable. Most retinal surgeons feel that if the retina has been attached longer than 6 months, the exoplant can be safely removed. Often, the motility abnormality is due to scarring and adhesions around the foreign material. In this case, additional manipulation can make matters worse, and removing the buckle rarely restores normal ocular motility. Leaving the buckle in place and working just on the involved muscle is usually more effective.

COMMENT

David A. Plager, MD

The eye and orbit were not designed to have bulky retinal hardware deflecting the course of the extraocular muscles or restricting motility by their bulk alone. In almost all cases, the bulky sponge or pillow should be removed, and the encircling element as well when possible. This gives the best chance to restore more normal motility and eliminates the problem of where to resuture the muscle when the hardware is in the way. As Dr. Buckley points out, most retinal surgeons agree that after 6 or at most 12 months, any retinal adhesion is complete and the buckle is no longer performing a necessary function.

2. *Adjustable sutures and hangback recessions:* In most strabismus situations caused by retinal surgery, some type of rectus recession is necessary. If the scleral band is left in position, it is often located at the site of the proposed recession. Several approaches can be used to overcome this problem. First, a marginal myotomy can be performed. This eliminates the need for sutures, but is somewhat unpredictable and makes for difficult reoperations. A second approach is to use a hangback recession, in which the muscle is "hung" from the original insertion site. This can be combined with the adjustable suture technique to maximize postoperative alignment. Nonabsorbable sutures can be used if subsequent reattachment to the globe is questionable. A third option is to combine a recession and resection of the same muscle and then suture the muscle behind the band or exoplant. A planned 5.0 mm recession could be converted to an 8.0 mm recession if a 3.0 mm resection is also performed. Very large recessions and resections will result in a faden-operation-like effect and should be avoided unless that is the desired effect.

COMMENT

Marshall M. Parks, MD

The sponge problem in dealing with restrictive strabismus for a retinal surgeon who insists that the sponge not be removed can be managed by a technique that disinserts the rectus muscle needing recession or advancement and passes it beneath the sponge that is in the way. Windows created in the sponge by excising enough to expose the scleral site for suturing the muscle without affecting its scleral compression are frequently used. Rectus muscles sutured to the encircling band do well, but I question whether hoping a hungback rectus muscle will attach itself to a sponge is the best selection.

3. *Surgery on the normal eye:* Careful consideration should be given to performing surgery on the uninvolved normal eye. Although most patients are hesitant at first, a careful explanation of the benefits of this approach often allays their fears. Even in situations in which a significant restrictive component exists, extraocular muscle surgery on the contralateral eye can be very successful and avoid the often unpredictable results associated with muscles involved in previous scarring and adhesions. Small vertical and horizontal deviations, especially when associated with mild incomitance, are often better handled with single muscle recessions on the uninvolved eye.
4. *Recession of conjunctiva and Tenon's tissue:* Care must be exercised in dealing with the conjunctiva and Tenon's tissue. During retinal detachment repair, extensive manipulation of these tissues occurs and accurate closure is often difficult, especially in older patients. The scarring that often results can be a factor causing restriction of eye movement. After strabismus surgery, consideration should be given to recessing this tissue to avoid creating a mechanical limitation. This is especially important in those situations where significant conjunctival adhesions were found and extensive dissection was required.

Surgical approach. Table 6–3 outlines the surgical approaches to correcting strabismus after retinal detachment surgery.

As mentioned earlier, vertical deviations are the most common type of strabismus causing diplopia. These deviations can be hypertropia, hypotropia, iatrogenic Brown syndrome, or cyclotropia.

1. *Hypertropia:* The usual surgical approach involves exploration of the offending fornix, paying careful attention to the position of the oblique muscles. For superior problems, careful dissection on both the nasal and temporal sides of the superior rectus is necessary because scar tissue and adhesions may make identification of structures difficult. If the superior oblique tendon is found trapped in this tissue, releasing the tendon and returning it to its normal anatomic position should be attempted. Forced duction testing before the conclusion of the operation is essential to ensure the elimination of any residual restrictive component.

   If a large exoplant under the superior rectus is suspected to be a source of the vertical deviation, it should be removed, and the superior rectus can be placed on adjustable suture. If removal of the exoplant is contraindicated, then a hangback superior rectus recession, with or without the adjustable suture technique, can be performed. A similar approach is used for inferior fornix restrictions, but downward restriction in this location is caused by the mass effect of the exoplant or adhesions to periorbital tissue rather than by tethering (Fig. 6–13).

Table 6–3 Treatment Strategies for the Involved Eye and/or the Contralateral Eye*

Presentation	*Cause*	*Ductions*	*Forced Ductions*	*Treatment of Involved Eye*	*Treatment of Contralateral Eye*
Horizontal	Visual loss	Normal	–	Recession/Resection	Recession/Resection
Comitant	—	—	—	—	—
Incomitant	Restriction (fat adherence)	Limited abduction	+	Recession MR ±resection LR	Recession MR Fadenoperation MR Resection LR
Hypertropia	Anteriorization of SO	Normal	–	Freeing SO tendon	—
	Superior restriction (exoplant)	Limited depression	+	Recession SR ± removal of exoplant	—
	Inferior restriction (exoplant)	Limited depression	+	Resection IR Removal of exoplant	Possible recession IR
Hypotropia	Inferior restriction (fat adherence)	Limited elevation ±depression	+	Freeing adhesions Recession IR ± resection SR	Possible recession SR or fadenoperation IR
	Inferior restriction (exoplant)	Limited elevation	+	Recession IR ± removal of exoplant	Possible recession SR
	Superior restriction (fat adherence)	Limited elevation	+	Freeing adhesions ±resection SR ±recession IR	Recession SR
	Superior restriction (exoplant)	Limited elevation	+	Resection SR Removal of exoplant	Possible recession SR
	Brown syndrome (iatrogenic)	Limited elevation (in adduction)	+	Freeing SO tendon	Recession SR
Cyclotropia	Anteriorization of SO	Normal	–	Freeing SO tendon ±Harada-Ito	Displacement SR/IR
	Anteriorization of IO	Normal	–	Freeing IO ± recession IO ± Harada-Ito procedure	Displacement SR/IR

*Surgery should be performed on the involved and/or the contralateral eye, depending on the amount of deviation and ocular rotations.

± = With or without; additional surgery as needed.

IO = inferior oblique; IR = inferior rectus; LR = lateral rectus; MR = medial rectus; SO = superior oblique; SR = superior rectus.

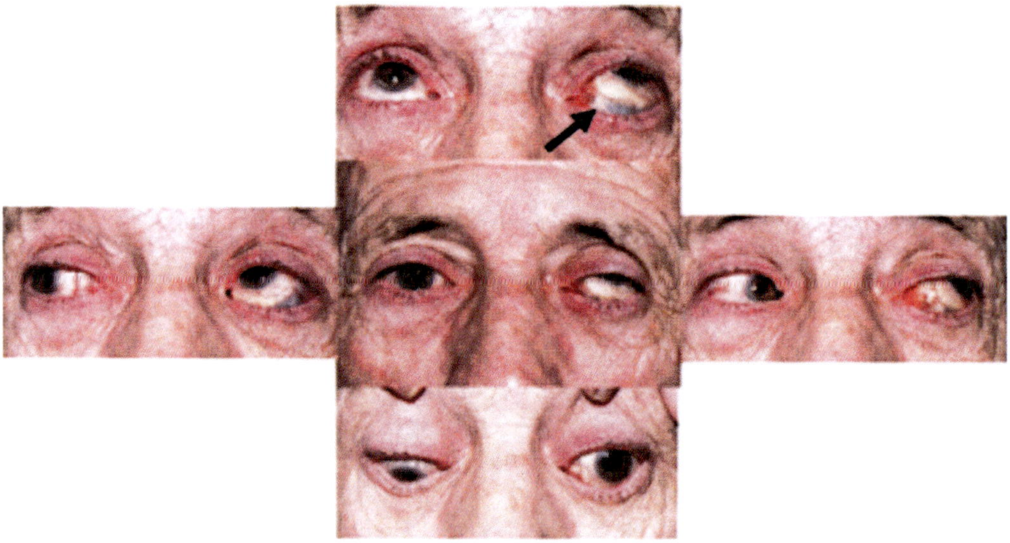

Figure 6–13. Large hypertropia due to an exoplant under the inferior rectus (*black arrow*).

2. *Hypotropia:* As with hypertropia, treatment for hypotropia involves exploration of the offending fornix, looking for adhesions or anterior placement of the oblique muscle. If there is a large exoplant under the inferior rectus, placing the rectus on adjustable suture or performing a hangback recession is usually necessary (Fig. 6–14). Removal of the exoplant is seldom sufficient to restore normal motility, though it can be helpful if a superior bulky exoplant is restricting upward movement (Fig. 6–15). The inferior oblique muscle or superior oblique tendon may also be anteriorized, contributing to a restriction in up gaze. Careful dissection along the lateral border of the inferior or superior rectus helps identify this situation. Adhesions should be

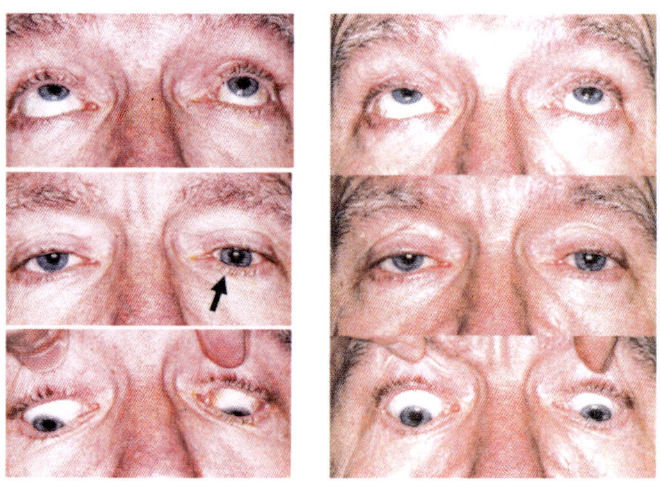

A B

Figure 6–14. (*A*) A scleral buckle on the left eye caused hypotropia (*black arrow*). (*B*) After a small recession of the left inferior rectus, the patient regained binocular function.

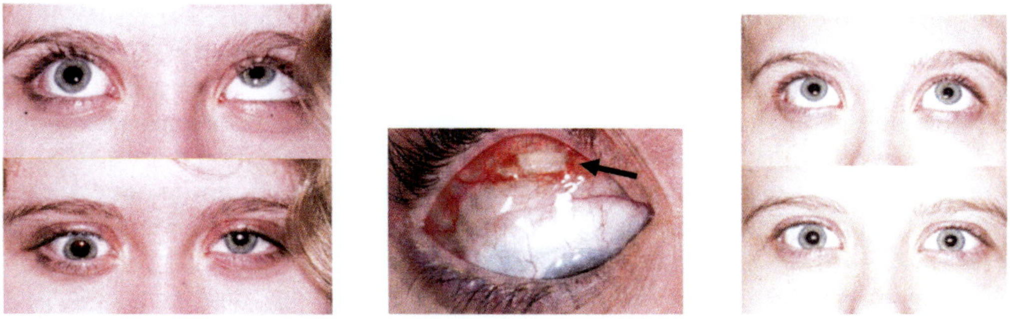

A B C

Figure 6–15. Retinal detachment surgery. (*A*) Hypotropia and inability to elevate the right eye after retinal detachment surgery. (*B*) Note the large exoplant eroding through the conjunctiva (*black arrow*). (C) The patient after removal of the exoplant and advancement of the superior rectus. Note the improved primary-position alignment and restored up-gaze movement of the right eye.

freed from the oblique muscle or tendon, and an attempt should be made to restore the oblique to its normal anatomic position, although this is seldom effective in an isolated procedure.

Treatment of inferior fat adherence is difficult. Although an effort should be made to release adhesions and scar tissue from the inferior rectus, this is usually not sufficient to restore normal ocular rotations. Forced duction testing before surgical intervention and at the conclusion is helpful in ascertaining whether significant restrictions have been eliminated. However, negative forced ductions do not ensure normal function postoperatively. Because of the difficulty in completely eliminating the restriction, it is usually necessary to recess the inferior rectus. Occasionally, this recession of the inferior rectus creates a new problem (hypertropia) on down gaze that can be addressed by surgery on the contralateral inferior rectus (faden-operation).

3. *Brown syndrome:* Incorporating the superior oblique tendon into the scleral band can cause a pseudo-Brown syndrome. Surgical exploration of the superior nasal quadrant and possible removal of the encircling band are necessary. Forced duction testing before completion of the surgical procedures is necessary to ensure that the restriction has been eliminated.
4. *Cyclotropia:* Excyclotorsion without a significant restrictive component can be improved by the modified Harada-Ito procedure. This involves lateralization of the anterior half of the superior oblique tendon and can be performed with the adjustable suture technique in a cooperative patient. Excyclotorsion can occur by changing the force vector of the superior oblique when it is trapped underneath the scleral buckle. In this circumstance, removing the buckle and returning the tendon to its normal position is usually sufficient. If the inferior oblique is tucked under the scleral band, a resultant hypotropia and excyclotropia secondary to tightening of the inferior oblique results. This can be treated by a myectomy of the inferior oblique.

Horizontal deviations are due to either sensory deprivation or restriction. If no restriction exists, treatment can be directed toward either eye with standard surgical techniques and amounts. In restricted situations, the surgeon must free the adhesions on the involved side or weaken the contralateral yoke muscles on the opposite eye by either recession or fadenoperation. A combination of esodeviation in one gaze direction with an associated exodeviation in the opposite direction indicates far posterior adhesions, and correction usually requires surgery on both eyes (Fig. 6–16).

As with vertical deviations, removal of the exoplant is rarely curative, and hangback recessions and adjustable sutures are quite useful. Resections should be used cautiously and should never be used as a single treatment strategy in patients with a restrictive horizontal component.

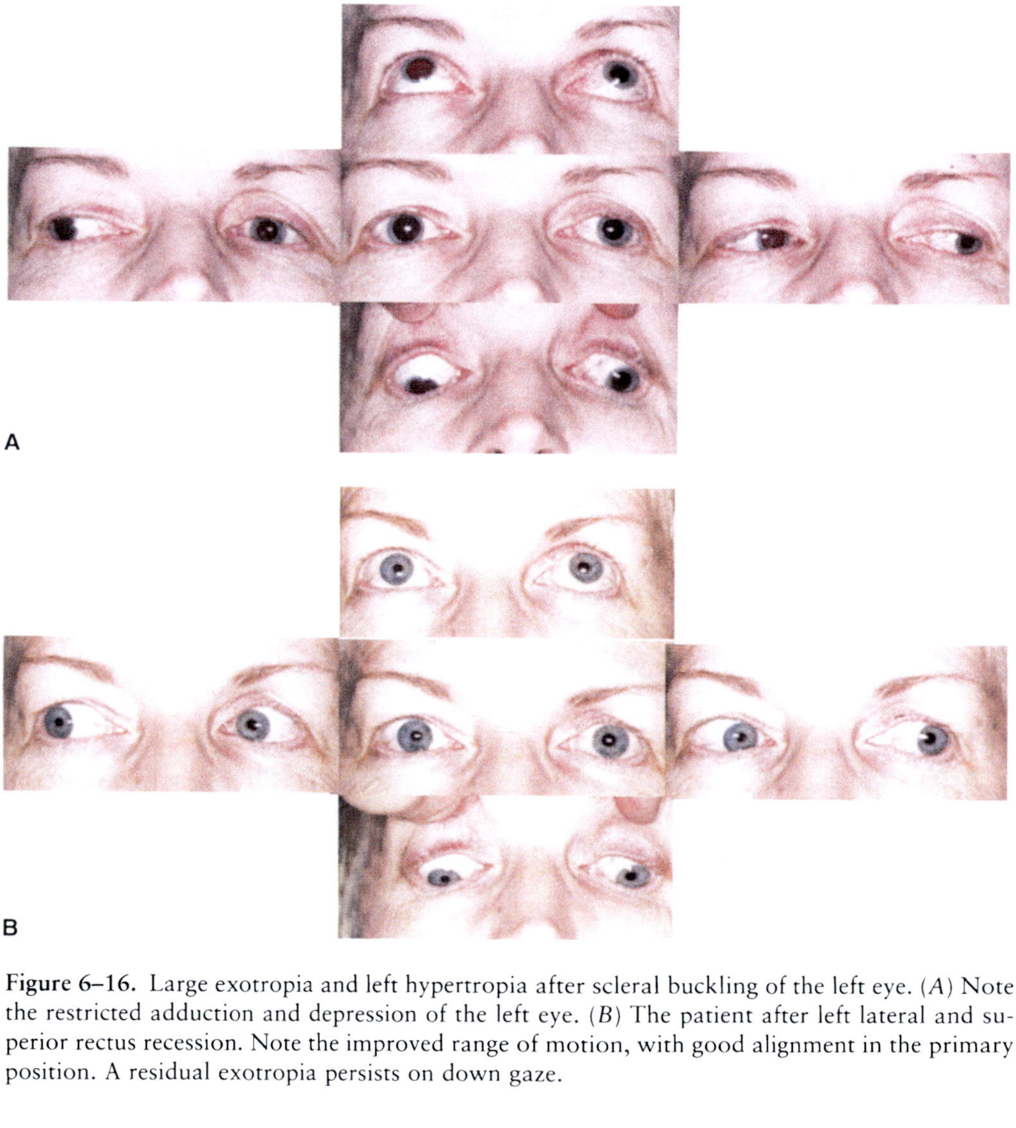

A

B

Figure 6–16. Large exotropia and left hypertropia after scleral buckling of the left eye. (*A*) Note the restricted adduction and depression of the left eye. (*B*) The patient after left lateral and superior rectus recession. Note the improved range of motion, with good alignment in the primary position. A residual exotropia persists on down gaze.

CATARACT SURGERY

Diplopia after cataract surgery can be caused by a preexisting strabismus, fusion loss due to deprivation, surgical trauma, or anesthetic myotoxicity. The first two causes do not normally have a restrictive component. In these situations, the vision loss associated with the cataract either masks or exacerbates the underlying motility disturbance. This is usually seen in cases with monocular cataracts or bilateral cataracts with significant differences in visual acuity. A preexisting strabismus, such as an intermittent exotropia, is made worse by the loss of vision associated with the cataract but is unrecognized because of the visual loss. Once the cataract is removed, the eye condition becomes apparent and the patient is diplopic. Other conditions, such as mild thyroid eye disease, cranial nerve palsies, or macular diseases, can present in a similar manner.

A restrictive strabismus can occur after cataract surgery and is currently thought to be caused by myotoxicity of local anesthetic agents or trauma to orbital tissues, nerves, and muscles. The exact mechanism by which local anesthetics injure extraocular muscles is not known. Studies have shown that when anesthetics are injected directly into extraocular muscles, extensive damage can occur, with loss of muscle fibers and the production of fibrous tissue. The susceptibility to muscle injury depends on the volume, concentration, and site of the injection and on the age of the patient.

Diagnosis. The motility abnormalities seen after cataract surgery fall into three general categories: contracture, overaction, and paresis.

1. *Contracture:* Contracture appears to be a direct result of injury from the anesthetic agents. In some circumstances, an initial paretic phase occurs, followed rapidly by fibrosis and tightening of the involved muscle. The final appearance is very similar to that seen in thyroid eye disease and often involves the inferior rectus. Some reports of undiagnosed thyroid myopathy as a cause of postoperative diplopia may have been due to this phenomenon. The contracture progresses rapidly and usually stabilizes by 4 to 6 weeks. Any of the extraocular muscles can be involved, although the vertical muscles are most commonly affected.
2. *Overaction:* A very common presentation looks like a childhood strabismus, with primary overaction of the involved muscle, such as the superior rectus, without any obvious weakness of the antagonist muscle (inferior rectus). In this situation, the patient has a large vertical deviation, but excellent movement and no restriction on forced duction testing (Fig. 6–17). This pattern of strabismus can be explained by a shift in the length tension curve, such as is seen after a small resection. Whether muscle contracture or overaction occurs depends on the degree of muscle fiber regeneration and eventual fibrotic proliferation. Mild fibrotic changes result in overaction, with more severe changes causing actual limitation.
3. *Paresis:* Occasionally, the involved muscle behaves as if it were paretic. On forced duction testing, there is neither limitation nor significant antagonist overaction. The cause is probably direct trauma or direct anesthetic toxicity

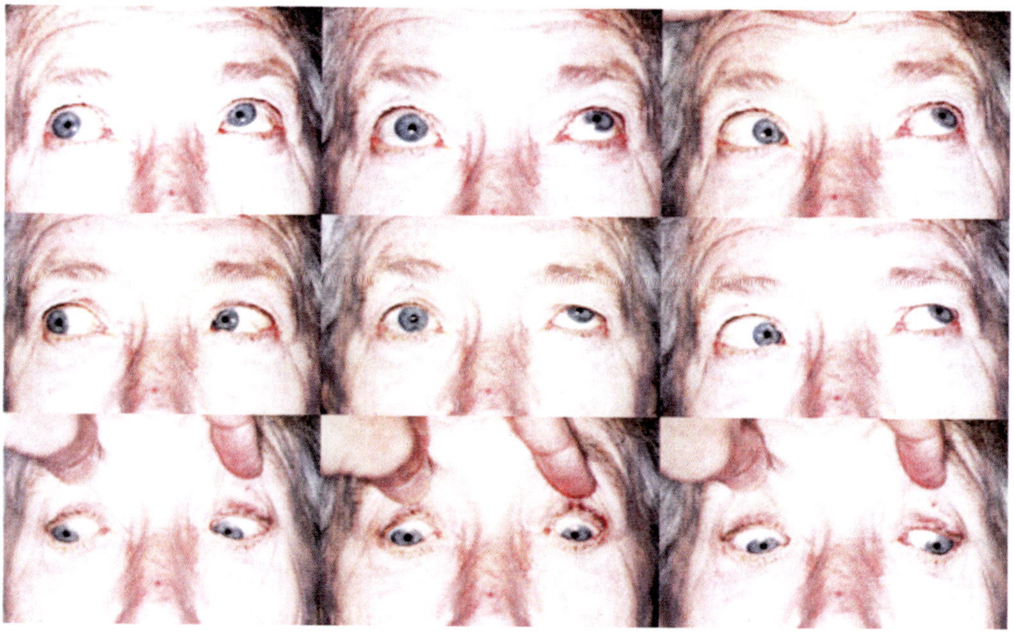

Figure 6–17. Overaction after cataract extraction of the left eye. Note the marked left hypertropia in the primary position, with no inferior rectus weakness. The left superior rectus markedly overacts on left gaze. Forced duction testing was negative.

to the extraocular muscle. This typically involves the inferior rectus and presents as a hypertropia with subnormal infraducting saccades.

Surgical Treatment. Most patients present with a vertical deviation and, regardless of the cause (contracture or overaction), the treatment is the same. Single vertical muscle recessions are generally used and can be combined with the adjustable suture technique (Fig. 6–18). Relatively large vertical deviations (20 to 25 prism diopters) can be treated with single recessions that typically are smaller than would be expected to be necessary. This is especially true with the overaction pattern. Rarely is it necessary to recess these vertical muscles more than 5.0 mm. In addition, postoperative incomitance occurs infrequently, and inferior rectus fadenoperations for residual down-gaze deviations are uncommon.

CONGENITAL FIBROSIS SYNDROME

Congenital fibrosis syndrome is a generalized restriction of extraocular muscles that classically presents with bilateral ptosis, marked limitation of up gaze, convergence on attempted up gaze, and limited horizontal eye movements. The patient often uses a chin-up head position to see at distance and may develop a head turn if horizontal alignment is severely affected. The cause is unclear, although increasing evidence supports a congenital defect in innervation that leads to progressive fibrosis of the extraocular muscles.

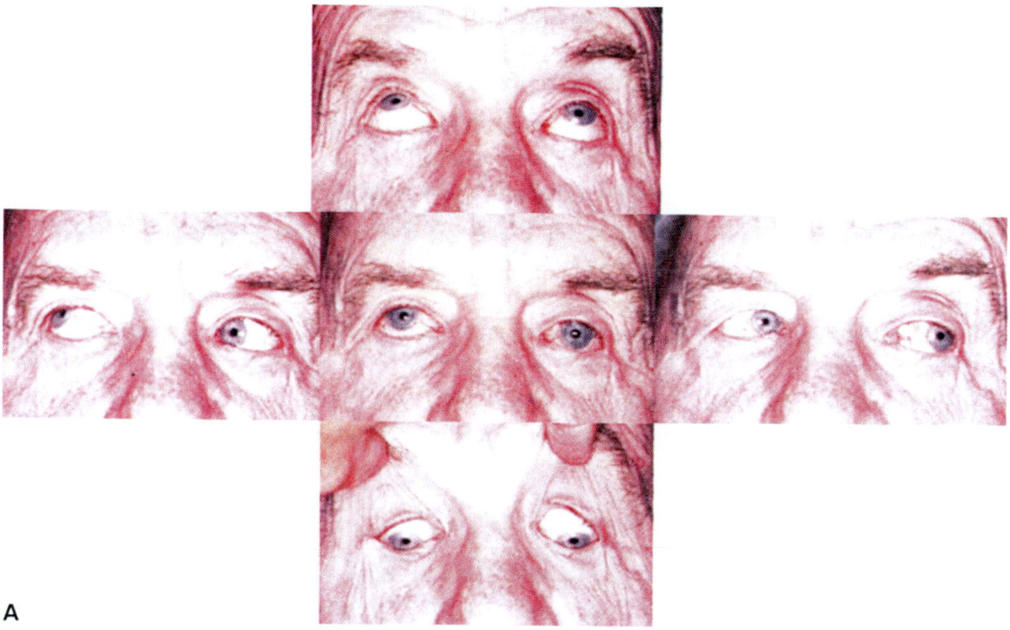

A

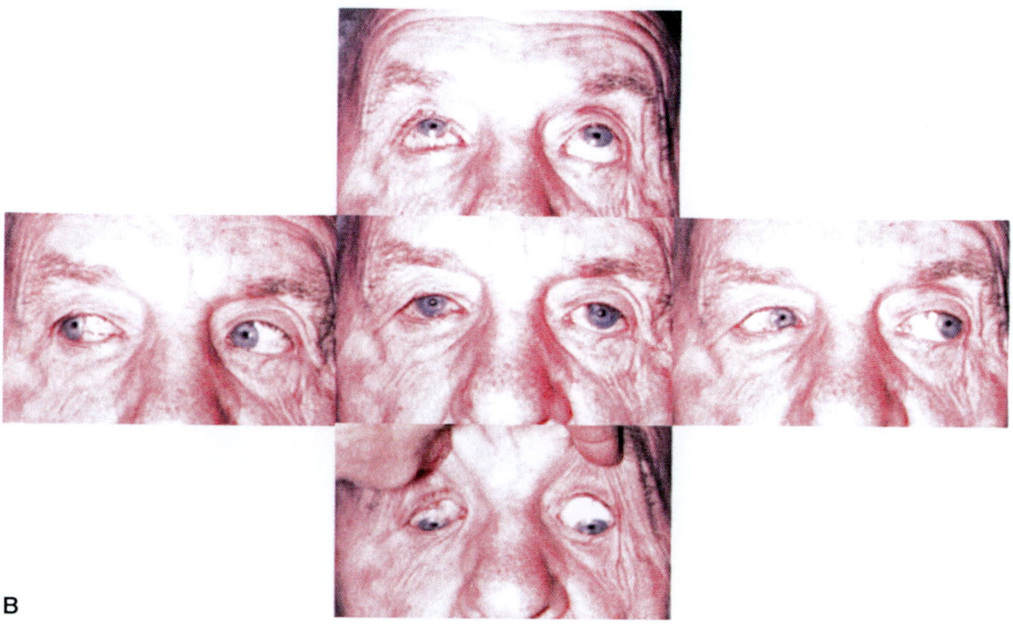

B

Figure 6–18. Large right hypertropia after cataract surgery with retrobulbar injection. (*A*) Note the marked overaction of the right superior rectus on right gaze. (*B*) Improved motility after right superior rectus recession, with restoration of single binocular vision.

The syndrome appears to be inherited as an autosomal dominant trait, with significant variability in the expressivity of the gene. The gene is located on chromosome 12, although the gene itself has not been identified. Patients with Prader-Willi syndrome can have a motility disturbance similar to that of congenital fibrosis syndrome that may be due to a defect on chromosome 15.

Clinical Presentation and Diagnosis. The clinical diagnosis is usually evident since most patients have a typical appearance, with ptotic lids and a chin-up head position (Fig. 6–19). Difficulties in diagnosis arise when the extraocular muscle involvement is mild, very asymmetric, or otherwise atypical. More subtle or unusual presentations may require forced duction testing to confirm the restrictive nature of the abnormality, and the final diagnosis may not be confirmed until surgery reveals small, thin, fibrotic muscles. Even though the condition is congenital, it may not be obvious until the child assumes an upright posture at age 4 to 6 months.

The patient typically maintains both eyes in downward rotation and shows moderate exotropia, with an inability to move the eyes well in any direction (Fig. 6–20). The inferior and lateral rectus muscles are usually the most severely affected, but all of the muscles are involved. An "A" pattern usually occurs with time because of the increasing weakness of the medial rectus muscles plus a convergence substitution, which results in an esotropia on attempted up gaze. Tight inferior rectus muscles alone may cause convergence on up gaze because of increased adductive effect.

Other motility disturbances have been described, ranging from mild elevation defects to marked bizarre motility presentations. The hallmark of all of these manifestations is the discovery of thin, fibrotic muscles at the time of surgery.

The ptosis is due to levator muscle fibrosis. Significant corneal exposure problems can occur if the eye is severely hypotropic and levator function is poor. In some individuals, levator function is preserved and the ptosis is due to the hypotropia (pseudoptosis). Several cases of Marcus Gunn jaw wink, a congenital neuronal misdirection syndrome, in combination with congenital fibrosis syndrome have been reported, lending support to the neurogenic theory of causation.

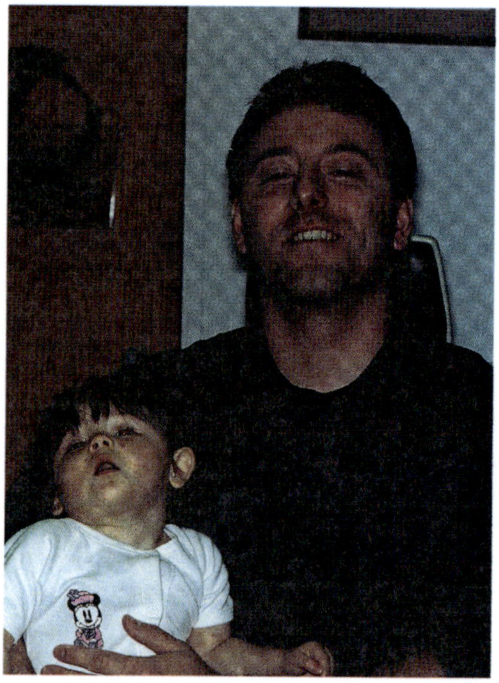

Figure 6–19. Father and daughter with congenital fibrosis syndrome. Both had significant elevation defects and adopted a chin-up gaze preference.

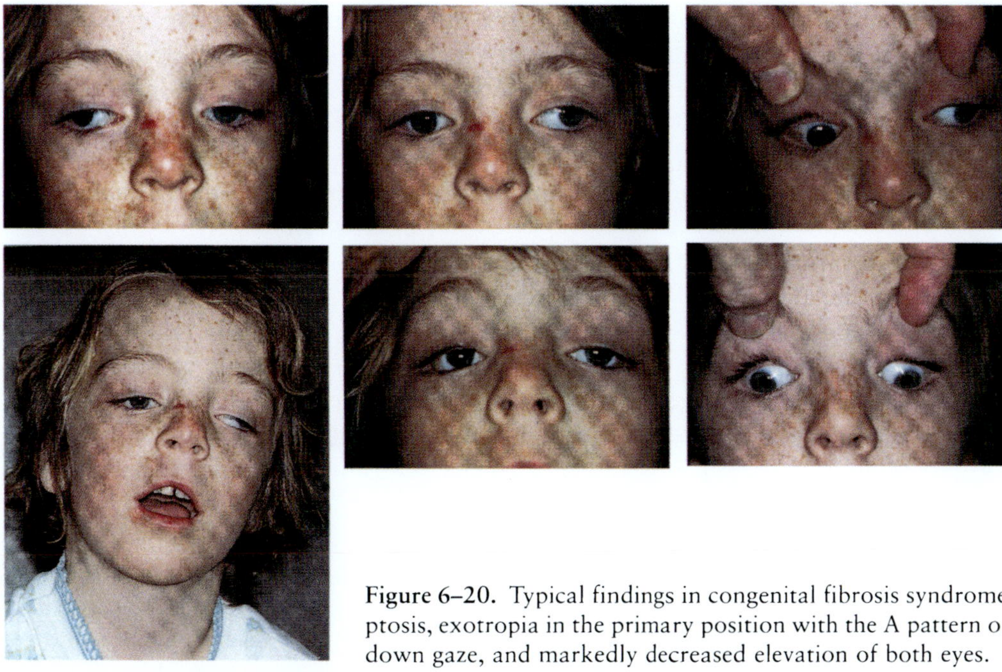

Figure 6–20. Typical findings in congenital fibrosis syndrome: ptosis, exotropia in the primary position with the A pattern on down gaze, and markedly decreased elevation of both eyes.

Differential Diagnosis. Any early-onset extraocular muscle or nerve abnormality can mimic congenital fibrosis syndrome. The most common ones are myasthenia gravis, double elevator palsy, third nerve palsy, and bilateral Brown syndrome. Differentiating these may be difficult, especially if the involvement is asymmetric (Table 6–4).

There are no specific tests for this disorder. Neuroimaging may be helpful in excluding other causes and can demonstrate thin, thread-like muscles, which are

Table 6–4 Differential Diagnosis of Congenital Elevation Deficiency

Condition	*Ptosis*	*Forced Ductions*	*Additional Muscles Affected*	*Pupil*	*Bell's Phenomenon*	*Horizontal Muscles Affected*
Congenital fibrosis syndrome	Yes	+	No Yes, if exotropia	No	No	Yes
Double elevator palsy	Pseudo or true	±	No	No	±	No
Myasthenia gravis	Yes	–	Yes	No	Absent	Yes
Third nerve palsy	Yes	–	Yes, medial rectus	±	Absent	Yes
Bilateral Brown syndrome	Pseudo	+	No	No	Present (±)	No

characteristic of this disorder. Probably the most important disorder to exclude is myasthenia gravis, since failure to identify it can have significant life-threatening consequences. In those patients with an obvious family history, no additional testing is warranted.

Surgical Treatment. The goals of therapy in this disorder are limited to placing the eyes in a functionally acceptable position. Unlike other restrictive strabismus conditions, restoration of useful ocular rotations is usually not possible because *all* of the muscles are involved. The standard approach of relieving the restriction still applies, but since there is no opposing force (that is, nothing is really being restricted), recessions are only moderately effective and serve only to shift the eye into a more usable position. Therefore, the aim of surgical intervention is limited to alignment in the primary position and down gaze, although even this may not be possible. The two most common problems requiring surgical intervention are hypotropia and exotropia.

1. *Hypotropia:* The inferior rectus muscles are preferentially involved in this disorder and are tight, fibrotic, and extremely thin. Care must be exercised during surgery to avoid tearing and fragmenting the muscles; thus, isolating and placing sutures can be quite challenging. In most circumstances, recession of the inferior rectus muscles improves the hypotropia, but even when completely detached from the globe, the eyes often remain hypotropic. The amount of recession required is substantial and at a minimum should be 6.0 to 7.0 mm (Fig. 6–21). Adjustable sutures are usually not necessary and, along with hangback recessions, may even be problematic. Since the opposing superior rectus muscles usually have little function, no real adjustment can be made and the muscle will reattach more anteriorly than desired if left hanging from the insertion. This can result in a substantial undercorrection.

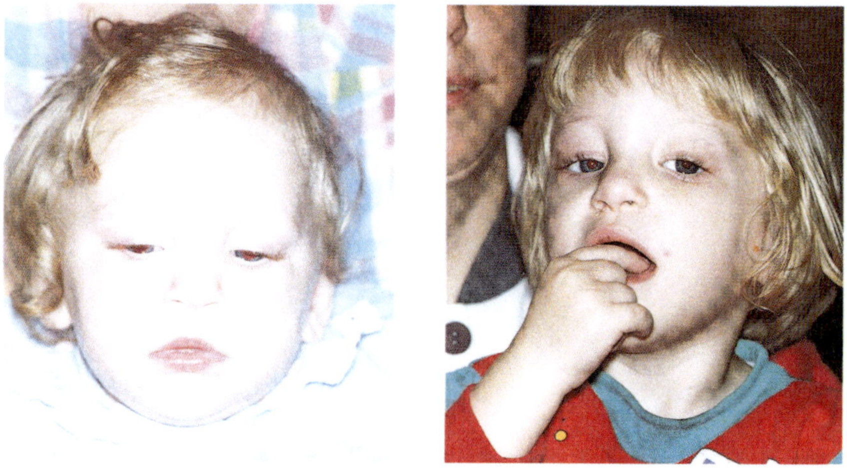

A B

Figure 6–21. Correction of hypotropia in congenital fibrosis syndrome. (*A*) Preoperative photograph of a young child with absent elevation of both eyes. (*B*) Same child after bilateral inferior rectus recessions. Note the slight residual chin-up head position, with ptosis and small exotropia.

To avoid this scenario, the muscle should be sutured to the eye, or the eye should be physically elevated with traction sutures for a short period of time postoperatively.

Resection of the opposing superior rectus will enhance the effect, but can severely limit down gaze and should be approached with caution. If the forced duction test reveals limitation of down gaze, then resection should be considered only if the deviation is marked. Even then, the amount of resection should be small (4.0 to 5.0 mm).

The goals of intervention are to raise the eyes just enough to reduce the chin-up head position necessary for distant viewing without severely limiting down-gaze functions such as reading. If ptosis is present, a very conservative frontalis sling may be necessary to avoid visual axis occlusion after surgery.

2. *Exotropia:* The exotropia seen in this syndrome is related more to medial rectus weakness than to lateral rectus fibrosis. Forced duction testing often reveals a global resistance to movement, yet a large exotropia is frequently present and becomes even larger on down gaze. To make matters worse, this A pattern is accentuated by an innervational abnormality, which results in convergence on attempted up gaze.

   Extremely large recessions of the lateral rectus muscles are necessary to improve this situation. As in recession of the inferior rectus muscles, the lateral rectus tendon should be sutured to the adjacent sclera to get the appropriate effect. Ideally, in most situations, the muscle should be detached completely since patients tend to end up undercorrected. Resecting the medial rectus can be attempted and is very powerful since it holds the eye in position, but it may worsen the convergence on up gaze. If medial rectus resections are performed, more conservative recessions of the lateral rectus are necessary to avoid marked overcorrections.

COMMENT

David A. Plager, MD

These patients, when severely affected, are usually undercorrected, no matter how large the inferior and lateral rectus recessions are. It is not unusual to have these patients return sooner or later for more surgery, which involves cutting the involved rectus muscles free from the eye and not reattaching them.

Suggested Readings

Aguirre-Aquino BI, Riemann CD, Lewis H, et al: Anterior transposition of the inferior oblique muscle as the initial treatment of a snapped inferior rectus muscle. *J Am Assoc Pediatr Ophthalmol Strabismus* 2001; 5:52–54.

Biesman BS, Hornblass A, Lisman R, et al: Diplopia after surgical repair of orbital floor fractures. *Ophthalmic Plast Reconstr Surg* 1996; 12:9–16; discussion 17.

Buckley EG, Meekins BB: Fadenoperation for the management of complicated incomitant vertical strabismus. *Am J Ophthalmol* 1988; 105:304–312.

Capo H, Guyton DL: Ipsilateral hypertropia after cataract surgery. *Ophthalmology* 1996; 103:721–730.

Christmann LM, Wilson ME: Motility disturbances after Molteno implants. *J Pediatr Ophthalmol Strabismus* 1992; 29:44–48.

Cruz OA: Restricted motility for vertical strabismus in Graves' ophthalmopathy. *Ophthalmology* 2001; 108:242–243.

de Faber JT, von Noorden GK: Inferior rectus muscle palsy after retrobulbar anesthesia for cataract surgery. *Am J Ophthalmol* 1991; 112:209–211.

Farr AK, Guyton DL: Strabismus after retinal detachment surgery. *Curr Opin Ophthalmol* 2000; 11:207–210.

Jaafar MS, Traboulsi, EI: Congenital fibrosis of the extraocular muscles. In: Rosenbaum AL, Santiago AP, eds: *Clinical Strabismus Management: Principles and Surgical Techniques*. Philadelphia: WB Saunders Co; 1999, 363–370.

Kushner BJ: Paresis and restriction of the inferior rectus muscle after orbital floor fracture. *Am J Ophthalmol* 1982; 94:81–86.

Seaber JH, Buckley EG: Strabismus after retinal detachment surgery: etiology, diagnosis, and treatment. *Semin Ophthalmol* 1995; 10:61–73.

Traboulsi EI, Jaafar MS, Hasan M. Kattan, et al: Congenital fibrosis of the extraocular muscles: report of 24 cases illustrating the clinical spectrum and surgical management. *Am Orthopt J* 1993; 43:45–53.

7

Nystagmus Surgery

MICHAEL X. REPKA

The decision to treat surgically a patient with nystagmus is a serious one. Such a plan is undertaken after considering each of the patient's symptoms and informing the patient and family of the likelihood of improvement.

INDICATIONS FOR SURGERY

Three symptoms lead the ophthalmologist to consider surgical correction of nystagmus: anomalous head posture, decreased vision, and oscillopsia. Surgery may also be performed for strabismus at the same operation.

1. Anomalous head posture, also called *ocular-induced torticollis*, is the most common symptom that is surgically treated. The patient positions the head so that the eyes are held in a direction of gaze in which there is minimal nystagmus (Fig. 7–1). This gaze position, called the *null position*, typically allows the optimal visual acuity, which can be measured in older children and adolescents. This demonstration can be useful when discussing the benefits of nystagmus surgery on the extraocular muscles. Surgical treatment does not eliminate the nystagmus, but repositions the null zone toward primary gaze.
2. Visual loss in patients with nystagmus may be due to the underlying abnormalities of the afferent visual system. Most children with congenital nystagmus have some type of sensory disorder, with estimates of prevalence ranging from 75% to 90%. The common causes include oculocutaneous albinism, optic nerve anomalies, and retinal abnormalities. Other patients may have no sensory defect and may be given a diagnosis of exclusion, commonly referred

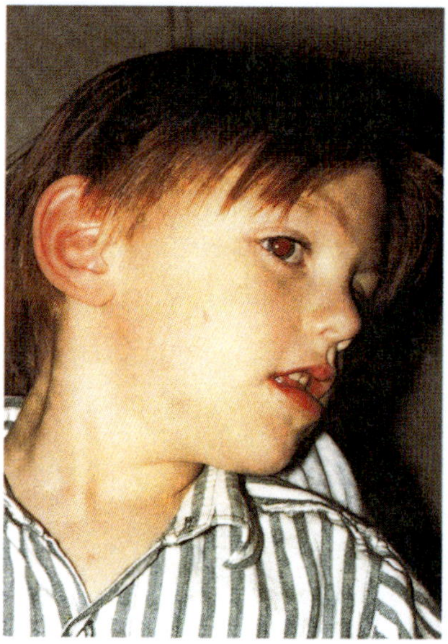

Figure 7–1. Anomalous head posture in congenital nystagmus.

to as *congenital motor nystagmus.* The continuous eye movements degrade the potential vision in both sensory and motor nystagmus.

3. The degradation of vision from the ocular movement also affects patients with acquired nystagmus. This latter group is further hampered by their recognition of either their eye movement or their relative environment movement, a symptom known as *oscillopsia.*

For both decreased vision and oscillopsia, the medical and surgical goals are to increase the foveation fraction (the portion of time the object of regard is on the fovea), which seems to be directly associated with best visual acuity. In general, surgical results for this indication have been modest.

PATIENT EVALUATION

The patient should undergo a comprehensive ophthalmologic history and examination. Careful evaluation for evidence of retinal or optic nerve pathology is needed. The eye movements should be observed carefully to be certain that there is no alternation of the fixation pattern or gaze preference. Electroretinography and neuroimaging may be needed if there is doubt about the cause of the nystagmus. If there is clinically significant refractive error, corrective spectacles should be provided. If the nystagmus is long-standing (for example, in an older child or an adult with onset in childhood), no additional workup is mandated. If the nystagmus is recently acquired or the history is unclear, neuroimaging is mandatory. Neurologic consultation may be useful to evaluate the patient with acquired nystagmus for evidence of a neurodegenerative condition.

Prior to an intervention, it is prudent to reexamine the patient after an interval of several months to be certain of the nature of the nystagmus. If eye movement recordings are available, they can be helpful in objectively evaluating the impact of therapy. (A comprehensive discussion of eye movement recordings and waveform analyses is beyond the scope of this book and is available elsewhere.)

BEHAVIORAL INTERVENTIONS

Parents and teachers need to be aware of any preferred head position and to be reminded that this is a useful adaptation and should not be discouraged. They should also ensure that vision is enhanced by making certain that the patient is positioned so that the chalkboard, teacher, television, and so on are in the favored direction of gaze. All too often, children have to accentuate the head turn because they are placed in the classroom on the side opposite to their zone of minimal intensity. For some patients, this is the only intervention they will need. In addition, since distance visual acuity is decreased relative to near acuity, it is not always apparent to the teacher that there is any visual problem. Adding this information to the school record can substantially aid a child's academic experience.

OPTICAL AND PHARMACOLOGIC INTERVENTIONS

Optical and pharmacologic interventions are not useful for anomalous head postures but can be helpful for patients with degradation of vision from the eye movements. The use of either rigid gas-permeable or soft contact lenses may damp the nystagmus of some patients, thereby increasing visual acuity. It is hypothesized that the sensory irritation from the contact lens leads to the improvement. As most of these patients are ametropic, this is a simple intervention to try, often with planned replacement-type soft contact lenses.

The most commonly prescribed medications for the management of congenital nystagmus have been baclofen and 5-hydroxytryptophan, both of which have had modest success. Clonazepam has been used for many types of acquired nystagmus. The benefit of improved visual acuity lasts for 2 to 6 hours. However, sedation is a side effect of this medication, limiting its usefulness for patients who work. The most widely used medication for eye movement disorders, including nystagmus, has been carbamazepine. Careful continuing hematologic and liver function testing is needed while a patient is being treated with this drug.

Botulinum Toxin. Botulinum neurotoxin A has been used by some clinicians to damp nystagmus and thereby reduce the symptoms of diminished vision and oscillopsia. This drug has been administered in one of two ways:

1. The first and most widespread method is the injection of 20 to 30 units into the retrobulbar space using a 25-gauge 30.0-mm needle.
2. The physician may selectively inject each of the horizontal rectus muscles with 2.5 to 5 units of botulinum toxin.

With both approaches, the amplitude of the nystagmus is markedly reduced. Ductions are only minimally impaired, and ptosis is remarkably uncommon. However, versions are markedly underactive, leading to troublesome diplopia. Thus, this method seems best suited for patients with significant visual loss (for example, optic neuropathy). In fact, some of the most satisfied patients have been those with demyelinating disease and reduced vision in one eye.

Some patients with nystagmus have found that botulinum treatment allows them to regain nearly normal visual acuity and resume normal activities. For most, the duration of treatment is 3 or 4 months. Patients with oculopalatal myoclonus after a brain stem infarct have been effectively treated with a single injection for as long as a year.

COMMENT

Edward G. Buckley, MD

In my experience, the usefulness of botulinum toxin in the treatment of nystagmus is extremely limited. Because of the significant motility disturbance that occurs after injection, binocular use is not beneficial. Injecting the botulinum toxin into the retrobulbar space causes a significant risk of ptosis, and the patient needs to be warned that manual lid elevation may be necessary. Since most of the acquired nystagmus patterns that can be treated with botulinum toxin have both a vertical and a horizontal component, functional improvement is often quite limited.

COMMENT

David A. Plager, MD

The (rare) prototype patient for whom retrobulbar botulinum is helpful is one with debilitating oscillopsia in one seeing eye from brain stem stroke. We treat a couple of such patients, one of whom has had more than 25 retrobulbar injections over a 7-year period. His acuity improves from 20/100 to 20/25 after the injection and remains 20/25 until the oscillopsia returns a few months later. We have learned through experience that ptosis can be prevented by having the patient sit upright immediately after the injection is given.

SURGERY FOR ANOMALOUS HEAD POSTURES

For more than a century, surgical therapy has been attempted for the relief of ocular abnormalities associated with nystagmus. Surgery has been most successful for the correction of anomalous head postures. It has also been used for patients in whom medical and optical approaches to the management of oscillopsia or reduced visual acuity have not been successful.

Surgery to eliminate an anomalous head posture involves moving the zone of minimal intensity (the null zone) toward the primary-gaze position, thus reducing the head turn. Surgery to improve visual acuity involves damping the motion of the eye, thereby increasing the foveation fraction and improving visual acuity.

There is no optimal time for this surgery. For the patient with a history of congenital nystagmus, it is probably best to wait until the patient is 4 or 5 years of age. The delay allows maturation of the binocular visual system. This should reduce the likelihood of a permanent iatrogenic strabismus and loss of binocularity following surgery. In patients with acquired nystagmus, it is important to wait at least 1 year after onset to allow evolution of the nystagmus waveform and the potential changes in head posture that could ensue.

Horizontal Anomalous Head Posture. The most common abnormal head posture associated with nystagmus is a horizontal turn to either the left or the right. The eyes are directed to the opposite side. The posture is most pronounced for finely detailed targets. Once the decision to offer surgical correction is made, it is important to measure the magnitude of head turn, as the surgery recommended is graduated. This can readily be done with an orthopedic goniometer (Fig. 7–2), although there are other sophisticated instruments such as helmet-based protractors and eye position trackers.

The most common operation performed is termed the *Kestenbaum-Anderson operation*. In this operation, the surgeon performs a series of graduated recessions and resections on each of the rectus muscles. The classical surgical amount guidelines were described by Marshall Parks as 5.0, 6.0, 7.0, and 8.0 mm. Each eye would receive the same total of 13.0 mm of surgery. For example, consider a patient who has a head turn to the left, with the eyes held in dextroversion (Fig. 7–3). The left eye, which is held in adduction, would undergo a 5.0 mm medial rectus recession and an 8.0 mm lateral rectus resection. The right eye would undergo a 7.0 mm lateral rectus recession and a 6.0 mm medial rectus resection.

However, many surgeons have found that surgery performed according to these guidelines frequently leads to undercorrection. Therefore, surgeons today perform *augmented classical Kestenbaum-Anderson procedures*. The augmented procedures take the classical numbers and add additional surgery based on the magnitude of the head turn (Table 7–1). For head turns of more than 20°, the classical numbers are increased by 40%. For angles up to and including 20°, the classical numbers are augmented by 20%.

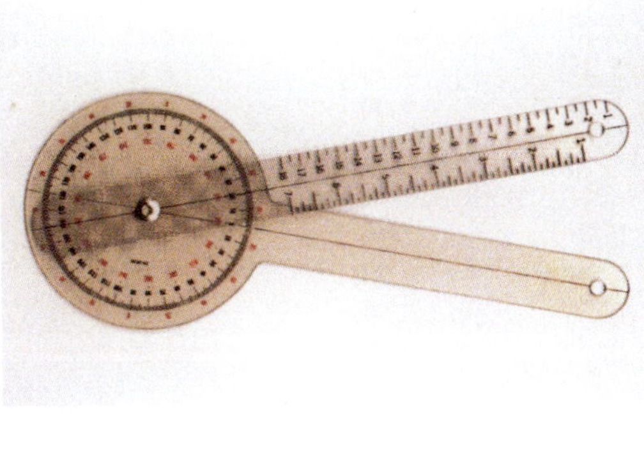

Figure 7–2. Orthopedic goniometer.

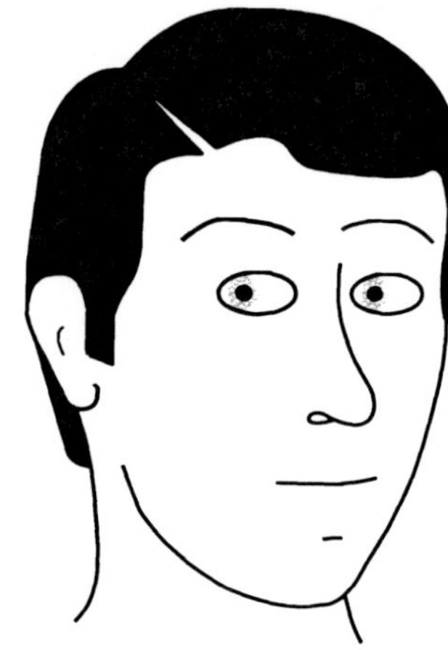

Figure 7–3. Kestenbaum-Anderson operation for anomalous head posture with left face turn would surgically move eyes to the left.

Eye movement recordings have been performed on just a few patients before and after they had this operation. These measurements have shown that the operation in the classic amounts will decrease the intensity of nystagmus in practically all gaze angles. The zone of minimal intensity is broadened and shifted toward the primary position.

This surgical procedure improves the head turn in a very high proportion of patients. Its success seems to be associated with a mechanical limitation of ductions away from the anomalous head posture. There are rare instances of overcorrection. Improvements in visual acuity are unusual and usually occur by only one line. However, nearly 40% of patients show evidence of recurrent head turn during long-term follow-up. Nevertheless, this procedure, particularly when done with the 40% augmented numbers, is successful in reducing the anomalous head posture.

Because of the difficulties with the Kestenbaum-Anderson procedure and the extensive amount of surgery performed, a reevaluation of the Anderson operation

Table 7–1 Surgical Amounts for Correction of Horizontal Anomalous Head Posture (mm)*

Magnitude of horizontal head turn	20°	21°–44°	45°
Right head turn: move eyes to right			
Recession right MR	6.00	6.50	7.00
Resection right LR	9.50	10.50	11.25
Resection left MR	7.25	7.75	8.50
Recession left LR	8.50	9.00	9.75
Left head turn: move eyes to left			
Resection right MR	7.50	7.75	8.50
Recession right LR	8.50	9.00	9.75
Recession left MR	6.00	6.50	7.00
Resection left LR	9.50	10.50	11.25

*Surgical amounts rounded to nearest 0.25 mm

LR = lateral rectus; MR = medial rectus.

of recessions only is in order. The classical recession numbers described by Anderson are inadequate. However, with enhanced surgical amounts, a 12.0 mm recession of the lateral rectus muscle and a 10.0 mm recession of the medial rectus muscle of the fellow eye improve the results. The theoretical advantages of the augmented Anderson operation are a reduced risk of anterior segment ischemia and the need to operate on only one muscle in each eye. Limiting surgery to one horizontal muscle in each eye is especially advantageous for the patient who may also need vertical rectus muscle surgery because of the presence of both horizontal and vertical torticollis.

COMMENT

Edward G. Buckley, MD

It has been my experience that recessions alone are not very effective in eliminating a head turn. Single-muscle recessions, even of large magnitudes, are usually ineffective over time; 1 to 2 years later, the head turn returns. In my experience, large resections, in combination with the weakening procedure, give a more stable permanent, long-term effect.

The surgeon considering nystagmus surgery should examine the patient more than once to be certain that the head posture is consistent over time. Numerous authors have commented on the unexpected overcorrection after surgery due to periodic alternating nystagmus. This pattern is found in both congenital and acquired forms of nystagmus, may have long periodicities, and is missed unless the patient is examined thoroughly over a long period of time. A Kestenbaum-Anderson or Anderson operation is ill advised in this situation. Instead, surgery recessing the four horizontal rectus muscles has been used with reasonable success (see the section "Surgery for Head Tilt").

COMMENT

Marshall M. Parks, MD

Kestenbaum applied a single number to each horizontal muscle in performing the bilateral recess-resect procedure for correcting the horizontal head posture the patient assumes to move the null point toward the primary position. The fallacy of using one number for all four horizontal muscles led me to choose the number for each muscle that in 1960 was considered the maximum that would not reduce the normal maximal duction excursion of the eye. Those numbers were 5.0 mm for recession of the medial rectus, 7.0 mm for recession of the lateral rectus, 6.0 mm for resection of the medial rectus, and 8.0 mm for resection of the lateral rectus. These numbers became known as the *classical amount*. The 13.0 mm of surgery performed on each eye evolved from the notion that "one size fits all," without consideration of the variation of the degree of abnormal head posture that occurs from patient to patient.

The classical numbers initially improved the head posture, but follow-up disclosed considerable return toward the preoperative status. The natural response was to increase the numbers, but on a scale according to the degree of malposition of the head: the classical amount plus 20%, 40%, and even 60%. As the numbers increased, the long-range outcomes correspondingly improved, but the downside was the reduction of the version amplitude manifest as the eyes attempted to turn in the opposite direction from which they were surgically moved. Hence, the conclusion became obvious: if the surgery was to be successful in managing the head posture, it had to be purchased at the price of a permanent reduction of the horizontal version amplitude in the direction of the preoperative abnormal head position.

My understanding of the neurophysiologic basis accounting for the two benefits resulting from the Kestenbaum or Anderson surgery is to center the null point toward the primary position without changing the innervational pattern to the extraocular muscles that obtunds the nystagmus excursions. The surgery blocks the movement of the eyes away from the primary position, while the same preoperative innervational pattern continues to the extraocular muscles that reduced the nystagmic excursions and permitted improved foveation time. When the null point is moved to the primary position, no longer is an unsightly and uncomfortable horizontal or vertical head posture necessary to achieve the best visual acuity.

COMMENT

Gunter K. von Noorden, MD

Occasionally, a severe face turn toward the side of the fixating eye develops in patients after enucleation or after severe loss of sight in one eye from disease or injury. This face turn is caused by an acquired jerky nystagmus with a null in adduction. In this situation, surgery on the fixating eye, consisting of recession of the medial and resection of the lateral rectus muscle, will normalize the head posture.

Coexistent nystagmus and strabismus. The examiner should measure the alignment, searching for any coexisting heterotropia. If there is a strabismus, it can be managed either in one step or as a staged procedure. First, the fixating eye must be determined. Moving this eye to the primary position should eliminate the head posture. Usually, the preferred or fixating eye is held in adduction, and a substantial medial rectus recession, coupled with a lateral rectus resection, is necessary.

If the surgeon has elected a staged approach, the surgery on the fixating eye is completed, while the surgery on the nonfixating eye is delayed for about 3 months. The strabismic deviation is measured before the second operation, and appropriate surgical amounts are planned. If a single-step procedure is planned, the surgeon may try to modify the surgical guidelines, based on the size of the concomitant esotropia or exotropia. A single-stage approach may be enhanced with adjustable sutures in the nonfixating eye.

COMMENT

Edward G. Buckley, MD

An even more difficult issue is how to approach the patient who has already had muscle surgery and requires additional surgery for the nystagmus with a residual strabismus. Again, Dr. Repka's general principle applies in aligning the fixating eye for the nystagmus and then making adjustments to the nonfixating eye for the strabismus. In most circumstances, if the patient is esotropic, less surgery will be required on the nonfixating eye than if the patient is exotropic. Since most of these patients have had previous surgery for esotropia (nystagmus block syndrome), the nystagmus surgery will be effective in correcting both the strabismus and the nystagmus. It is often necessary to operate only on the fixating eye or, at most, on one additional muscle on the nonfixating eye.

Vertical Anomalous Head Posture. Vertical head posture induced by nystagmus may manifest with either a chin-up or a chin-down position. A vertical posture is less common than a horizontal posture, although it may also be combined with a horizontal posture. In patients with both horizontal and vertical components, it is usually advisable to treat the horizontal deviation first. In some cases, the resultant vertical posture is sufficiently minimized to obviate surgery. The operative plan should not include recession of all vertical and horizontal rectus muscles because of the risk of anterior segment ischemia.

The techniques for managing vertical postures are similar to those discussed for horizontal postures. However, the oblique muscles provide a surgical option for correcting vertical postures. The basic technique is to rotate the eyes surgically in the direction of the head turn. This would include a resection of the rectus muscles in the direction of the head posture and a recession of the yoke rectus muscles.

Just as with surgery for horizontal anomalous head postures, early surgical amounts of 4.0 and 5.0 mm were insufficient to achieve adequate results. Recessions of 7.0 mm for the superior rectus muscles and resections of 8.0 mm for the inferior rectus muscles are reported to produce excellent correction of chin-down postures. For chin-up postures, similar procedures involving resections of the superior rectus muscles and recessions of the inferior rectus muscles can be performed.

Alternatively, for chin-down posture a superior rectus recession might be combined with inferior oblique anteriorization, in which the inferior oblique is placed at the temporal edge of the inferior rectus muscle insertion. This modification may be particularly useful for patients in whom horizontal surgery is planned, because it allows the inferior rectus to remain unoperated. Head postures of 25° require surgery of at least 6.0 mm on all four vertical rectus muscles. For vertical torticollis greater than 25°, surgery of at least 7.0 mm on the four vertical rectus muscles is recommended.

COMMENT

Edward B. Buckley, MD

For vertical nystagmus, care must be exercised not to overresect the inferior rectus muscle. This can often result in lower lid elevation, which can be both functionally and cosmetically unacceptable. Resections greater than 6.0 mm should be done with caution because of this problem. Likewise, excessive recessions of the superior rectus, in combination with large resections of the inferior rectus, can result in marked upper lid elevation, which may have to be treated with levator recessions. Patients should be warned of this possibility.

SURGERY FOR HEAD TILT

A small number of patients have a nystagmus that induces a head tilt. These patients learn that by rotating the fundus relative to the environment, they may reduce the intensity of the nystagmus. Surgery is designed to re-create the preferred cyclotorsion when the head is held upright.

Surgery to correct abnormal ocular torsion induced by nystagmus may be accomplished by weakening or tightening the oblique muscles. Such muscle surgery directly affects the torsional state. It may also be done by using offsets of either the horizontal or the vertical rectus muscles; alternatively, a combination of rectus and oblique muscle surgery may be used. Surgery on the oblique muscles may run a greater risk of inducing a heterotropia. In any procedure, extra care must be taken to be certain that the planned surgery will produce the anticipated change in ocular position relative to the environment.

This author prefers offsets of the vertical rectus muscles. The tendon is shifted one full tendon width and reattached to the globe, maintaining the same distance from the new insertion to the limbus that was present preoperatively. These procedures typically involve two vertical rectus muscles in each eye. For instance, a head tilt to the left induces an incyclorotation of the right eye and an excycloration of the left eye relative to the environment (Figure 7–4). The surgical procedure must produce exactly the same result, so the patient no longer has to tilt the head to achieve the necessary torsion. In the right eye, incyclorotation is achieved by a temporal transposition of the right superior rectus and a nasal transposition of the right inferior rectus. In the left eye, excyclorotation is achieved by a nasal transposition of the left superior rectus and a temporal transposition of the left inferior rectus.

COMMENT

Gunter K. von Noorden, MD

A good way of remembering which direction to shift the eyes to treat an abnormal head posture secondary to nystagmus is: Move the eyes in the same direction as the head position. For instance, when the face is turned to the

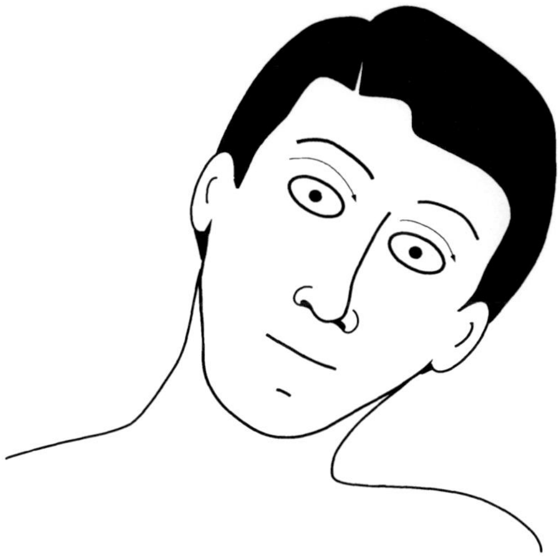

Figure 7–4. Surgical procedure for left head tilt. Extort the left eye and intort the right eye.

right, both eyes are shifted to the right. With a head tilt to the right shoulder, both eyes are rotated to the right around the visual axis; that is, the right eye is surgically extorted and the left eye is intorted.

Other surgeries for torsion have been described, but very little outcome data are available on this group of procedures:

1. Transpositions of the horizontal rectus muscles have been used. This procedure is similar technically and theoretically to the vertical muscle procedure. To create an excyclorotation, the lateral rectus muscle is moved up and the medial rectus muscle is moved down.
2. Another proposed procedure, although more complicated technically, is the advancement and recession of the oblique muscles. To produce an excyclorotation, the superior oblique is recessed and the inferior oblique muscle is resected and reattached to the globe.
3. A third procedure involves slanting the insertions of all the rectus muscles, with the recession on the side of the muscle to which the surgeon intends the eye to rotate.

COMMENT

David A. Plager, MD

The idea of performing torsional surgery on the four oblique muscles is theoretically pleasing but not very practical. Advancing or resecting the inferior oblique is particularly unfamiliar to most surgeons, and tucking or resecting an otherwise normal superior oblique tendon is likely to cause a Brown syndrome. The horizontal offsets of the vertical rectus muscles are easier, more predictable, and less troublesome.

SURGERY FOR VISUAL ACUITY

Surgery to improve visual acuity in the setting of nystagmus has been performed for more than half a century. Concerning this surgical therapy, periods of great excitement have alternated with periods of great disillusionment. No large series of patients or any randomized clinical trials have evaluated this treatment.

The most commonly performed surgery is a recession of all four horizontal rectus muscles. Such surgery has been found to improve visual acuity by approximately one line, although qualitative results have been better. The lateral rectus muscle should be recessed 10.0 mm from the insertion and the medial rectus about 7.5 mm from the insertion. Larger recessions of the medial rectus tend to lead to consecutive exotropia. This procedure is also valuable in the management of the alternating anomalous head postures associated with periodic alternating nystagmus.

COMMENT

David A. Plager, MD

> Rather than using preordained amounts of horizontal muscle recession in the four-muscle recession procedure, we have found it valuable to first recess either medial rectus (in a straight-eyed patient) to a point that can be safely reached and is posterior to the equator as the eye is visualized intraoperatively. That point is measured and is typically 13.0 to 17.0 mm from the limbus. The distance from the limbus can vary, depending on the age of the patient, the size of the eye, and other factors. The lateral rectus is then recessed a distance 2.0 mm greater from the limbus than the medial was—for example, 15.0 to 19.0 mm. This disparity prevents the consecutive exotropia that often develops if the medial and lateral rectus muscles are recessed by identical amounts. The same procedure is performed on the other eye.

Another surgical approach for the management of reduced visual acuity due to nystagmus is the creation of surgical or optical artificial divergence. Such a procedure may be considered for patients with binocular fusion. Preoperatively, base-in prisms are placed before the eyes, inducing an exotropia, which must be compensated for by convergence. Prism is increased until there is no additional improvement of visual acuity and the patient continues to fuse. The amount of prism represents the surgical angle and the amount of surgery. Either a single medial rectus recession of the preferred eye or, preferably, a combination with a medial rectus recession of the nonpreferred eye can be performed. About one in four patients will experience mild visual acuity improvement, and 10% or more will develop an exotropia.

COMPLICATIONS OF NYSTAGMUS SURGERY

No surgery is immune from complications. Three important complications of the procedures discussed in this chapter are as follows:

1. With all of the procedures, there is a chance of creating a heterotropia.
2. Many patients with nystagmus may eventually require surgery on all of their rectus muscles, leading to the chance of anterior segment ischemia.
3. All of these procedures are associated with a significant chance of undercorrection. Care should be taken to avoid overly optimistic forecasts of the expected outcomes.

COMMENT

Gunter K. von Noorden, MD

Dr. Repka mentions that there is a chance of creating a heterotropia with many of the surgical procedures for nystagmus. This statement is basically correct, but the risk is almost negligible and should not deter one from considering surgery for an abnormal head posture that has an excellent chance of being cured or improved by an operation. The only time I have seen heterotropia after nystagmus surgery was years after equal amounts of equally large recessions (10.0 mm) of all four horizontal rectus muscles had been performed to reduce the amplitude of nystagmus. An exodeviation developed, which responded well to a 3.0 mm advancement of the recessed medial rectus muscles. We did not encounter this problem again after we learned from this experience to recess the medial rectus muscles 2.0 mm less than the lateral rectus muscles during the procedure.

Suggested Readings

Flynn JT, Dell'Osso LF: The effects of congenital nystagmus surgery. *Ophthalmology* 1979; 86:1414–1427.

Helveston EM, Ellis FD, Plager DA: Large recession of the horizontal recti for treatment of nystagmus. *Ophthalmology* 1991; 98:1302–1305.

Hertle RW, Maldanado VK, Maybodi M, et al: Clinical and ocular motor analysis of the infantile nystagmus syndrome in the first 6 months of life. *Br J Ophthalmol* 2002; 86: 670–675.

Lee J: Surgical management of nystagmus. *J R Soc Med* 2002; 95:238–241.

Leigh RJ, Zee DS: *The Neurology of Eye Movements*. Philadelphia: FA Davis; 1991.

Repka, MX: Nystagmus: clinical evaluation and surgical management. In Rosenbaum AL, Santiago AP, eds: *Clinical Strabismus Management: Principles and Surgical Techniques*. Philadelphia: WB Saunders Co; 1999, 404–420.

Repka MX, Savino PJ, Reinecke RD: Treatment of acquired nystagmus with botulinum neurotoxin A. *Arch Ophthalmol* 1994; 112:1320–1324.

Roberts EL, Saunders RA, Wilson ME: Surgery for vertical head position in null point nystagmus. *J Pediatr Ophthalmol Strabismus* 1996; 33:219–224.

von Noorden GK: *Binocular Vision and Ocular Motility: Theory and Management of Strabismus*, 5th ed. St Louis: CV Mosby Co; 1996.

von Noorden GK, Jenkins RH, Rosenbaum AL: Horizontal transposition of the vertical rectus muscles for treatment of ocular torticollis. *J Pediatr Ophthalmol Strabismus* 1993; 30:8–14.

8

Reoperation Strategies

DAVID A. PLAGER

After strabismus surgery, a reoperation may be needed due to undercorrection, overcorrection, or a new strabismus problem that may or may not be related to the prior surgery. Rates of reoperation are difficult to determine and are related to myriad factors, including the complexity of the original problem, the patient's level of binocular sensory function, the patient's age, the development of new problems related to either the original surgery or the underlying diagnosis, and the skill and experience of the surgeon.

For instance, in long-term follow-up of operations performed at one medical center, the reoperation rate for superior oblique palsy was in the 10% to 20% range, depending on whether the patient had been previously operated on before referral, whereas the reoperation rate for congenital esotropia over a 10-year postoperative period was 120%. Put another way, superior oblique palsy patients, who tend to be older and have high-grade or normal fusional ability, needed 1.1 to 1.2 surgeries on average to correct their strabismus. By contrast, infants with congenital esotropia, who have subnormal binocular sensory systems, and are at risk for developing associated problems such as dissociated vertical deviations and oblique muscle dysfunction, required an average of 2.2 surgeries over the first 10 years postoperatively.

REOPERATION PRINCIPLES

The need for reoperation may become apparent soon after surgery or not until many years later. Challenges presented by reoperation raise the level of complexity for surgical planning and execution, and these procedures do not lend themselves to the surgical doses found in tables. There is no substitute for wide experience as the best teacher for coping with the limitless number of clinical scenarios that can be encountered in strabismus reoperations. However, there are a number of general principles for reoperation that can be applied.

Factors to consider in planning for reoperation include the following:

1. The history of the procedures done previously and for what condition(s) (if known)
2. The patient's present motility measurements, preferably in primary, up, down, and side gazes, as well as the near deviation
3. A careful assessment of ductions and versions, with emphasis on documentation of any muscle underaction or overaction
4. If any underaction is found, an assessment of generated force and forced ductions, the latter either preoperatively or intraoperatively, to determine whether the limitation is due to restriction

REOPERATION FOR RESIDUAL OR CONSECUTIVE HORIZONTAL STRABISMUS

Residual Esotropia After Esotropia Surgery. If horizontal versions are full, the patient can be treated as an essentially new case. The question is: Should the medial rectus muscles be re-recessed or the lateral rectus muscles resected, or should each be done on one eye? If the surgeon chooses to operate on the previously unoperated eye or muscle, conventional surgical dosage tables can be consulted. If the near esotropic deviation exceeds the distance deviations, the medial rectus recessions should be maximized prior to contemplating lateral rectus resection.

If the medial rectus has already been recessed 6.0 mm or more from the insertion, there is little to be gained from further recession without creating an adduction deficiency and an eventual consecutive exotropia. Lateral rectus resections would be indicated.

Consecutive Exotropia After Esotropia Surgery. The critical examination finding to look for is *any* limitation of adduction in an eye that has had previous medial rectus recession. This finding frequently indicates a slipped medial rectus or, at the least, an overly recessed medial rectus (Fig. 8–1). A deficient adduction could also result from a previous too large lateral rectus resection. In such cases, history can be a helpful guide. If the consecutive exodeviation follows medial rectus recession, any adduction deficit requires exploration and advancement of the true skeletal muscle of the medial rectus. If the medial rectus recession resulted in residual esotropia, which then required lateral rectus resection, any resulting exodeviation is probably best corrected by recession of the lateral rectus muscle(s) (Fig. 8–2).

In long-standing consecutive exotropia from any cause, the lateral rectus can become contracted and require recession. If horizontal versions are full, consecutive exotropia can be repaired by any combination of lateral rectus recession or medial rectus resection or advancement in one or both eyes that is appropriate for the preoperative deviation.

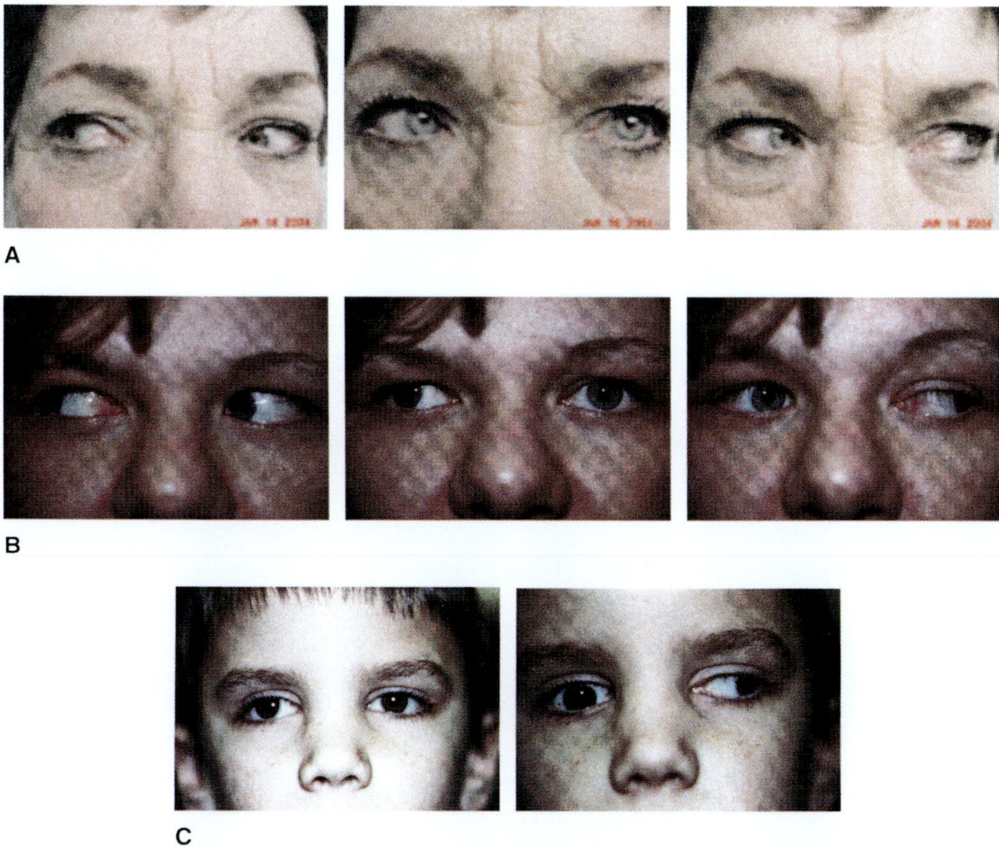

Figure 8–1. Adduction after medial rectus recession. (*A*) Full adduction bilaterally in residual esotropia. (*B*) Full adduction in the left eye and moderate limitation to adduction in the right eye in consecutive exotropia. (*C*) Marked limitation to adduction in the right eye in consecutive exotropia.

COMMENT

M. Edward Wilson, MD

When medial rectus muscles are advanced for long-standing consecutive exotropia, the effect is often less per millimeter than expected. When in doubt, the surgeon should advance the muscle all the way back to its original insertion. The relative tightness of the muscle in that advanced position is a good indication of the amount of exotropia that has been corrected.

COMMENT

Edward G. Buckley, MD

A common clinical scenario involves the patient with a fairly large-angle congenital esotropia who undergoes bimedial rectus recessions and later unilateral or bilateral lateral rectus resections for a significant residual esotropia. Years later, the patient develops an exodeviation with an apparent

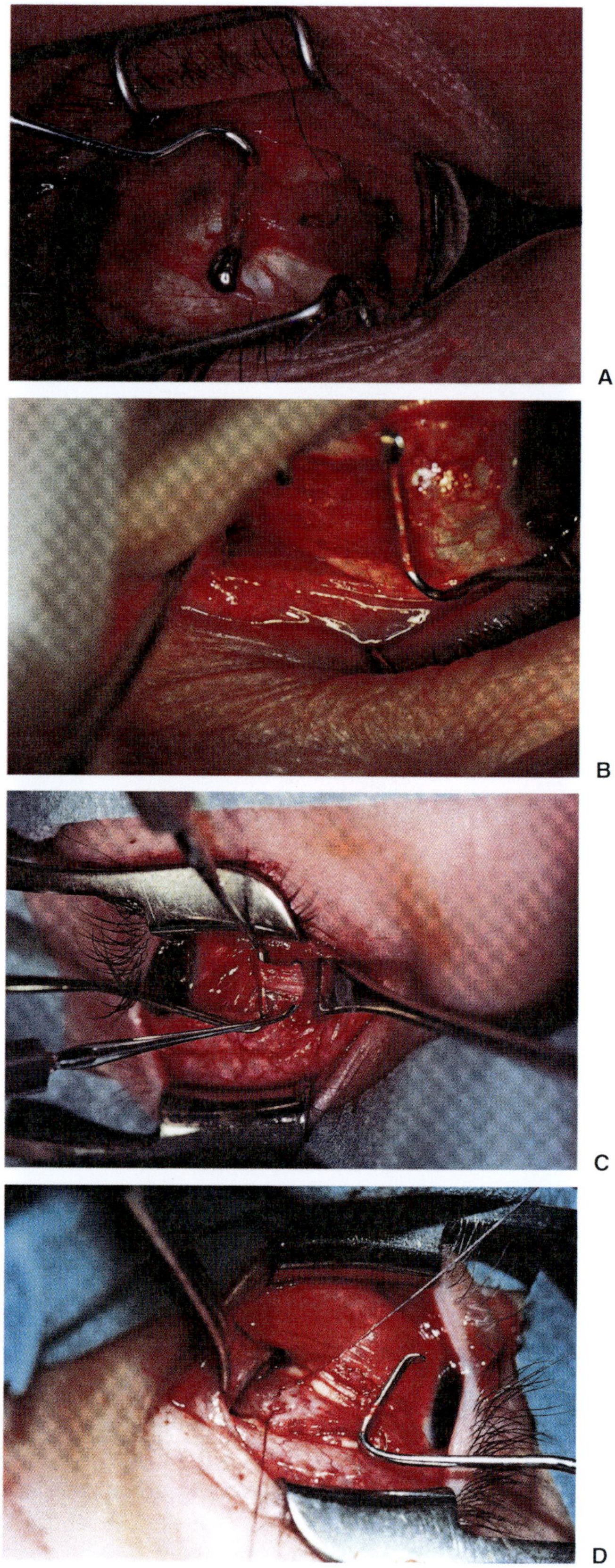

Figure 8–2. Slipped medial rectus. (*A*) Intraoperative photograph. The skeletal muscle portion shows fusiform expansion immediately posterior to the demarcation line between the empty capsule and the muscle. (*B*) Slipped muscle with a thin, translucent capsule through which the shine of the muscle hook can be seen. (*C*) Another slipped muscle with a thick, fibrotic empty capsule. (*D*) Repair of a slipped muscle requires that the muscle be secured with solid locking suture bites in skeletal muscle as shown. Nonabsorbable sutures are not necessary; the key to successful repair is securing solid muscle to the globe.

weakness of adduction of one or both eyes. Depending on the size of the deviation, simply advancing the weak medial rectus will be insufficient to eliminate the deviation. In this circumstance, both the weak medial rectus and the resected lateral rectus need to be addressed.

Residual Exotropia After Exotropia Surgery. If versions are full, the patient can be treated as if previously unoperated. The easiest and most predictable surgery would involve operating on the previously unoperated eye or muscle using conventional surgical dosages to recess the lateral rectus or resect the medial rectus. If this is not possible or preferable, as might be the case in a patient with only one good-seeing eye, re-recession of the lateral rectus up to 9.0 mm from the original insertion or re-resection of the medial rectus is the viable choice.

In a patient who is a candidate for surgery on both eyes, the lateral rectus muscles should be recessed (re-recessed) up to 9.0 mm from the insertion, and any residual deviation corrected by an appropriate amount of resection of one or both medial rectus muscles. If a patient has already had a lateral rectus recessed 7.0 mm or more, attention should be directed to medial rectus resection.

Consecutive Esotropia After Exotropia Surgery. In a fusing adult patient, consecutive esotropia after surgery for exotropia is likely to cause diplopia, and, in a child, development of suppression. If the consecutive esotropia lasts for more than a couple of weeks, it is important to prescribe prism spectacles to compensate for the deviation or, at least, to institute alternate patching to prevent suppression and remediate any diplopia.

COMMENT

Gunter K. von Noorden, MD

When consecutive esotropia occurs after surgery for exotropia and slippage of the lateral rectus muscle is not suspected, one of the first steps to be taken is to correct a previously uncorrected hypermetropia. Correction of even small amounts of hypermetropia may be useful in such patients, especially in those with a high accommodative convergence/accommodation (AC/A) ratio. To identify these patients preoperatively, we measure the deviation at near fixation with and without +3.00 spherical lenses.

COMMENT

Michael X. Repka, MD

I generally wait at least 6 months with prism correction in place before undertaking a second surgery. Because the delayed outward drift back toward an exodeviation is very common, it makes sense to wait before having the patient undergo another operation. There would be a very high chance of restoring the patient to an exodeviation.

Once the permanence of the consecutive esotropia is established and reoperation is planned, concerns similar to those described above for consecutive exotropia should be considered. Specifically, if there is any limitation of abduction associated with consecutive esotropia, medial rectus restriction should be ruled out by forced ductions or treated by recession. Alternatively, if forced ductions are free, the offending lateral rectus must be explored to rule out and repair any slipped muscle.

If all horizontal ductions are full, consecutive esotropia can be treated by recession of one or both medial rectus muscles—both if the deviation is greater than 15 prism diopters. An esotropia greater at distance than at near is an indication to advance or resect previously recessed lateral rectus muscles rather than recess the medial rectus muscles.

COMMENT

M. Edward Wilson, MD

Consecutive esotropia with full ductions (the surgeon should look carefully for lateral rectus muscle weakness) can be treated with medial rectus muscle recessions (fresh muscles) or with lateral rectus muscle advancements (Cooper's dictum). I think this is true even if the esotropia is greater at distance, provided that the lateral rectus muscle ductions are normal. There is no proof that lateral rectus surgery has more effect at distance than at near.

REOPERATION FOR NEW VERTICAL DEVIATION

If the patient has not developed a coincidental vertical muscle problem, such as third or fourth nerve palsy, thyroid disease, trauma, or dissociated vertical deviation, a new vertical deviation must be assumed to be iatrogenic. A careful observation of versions, followed by forced ductions, will likely reveal a relative restriction in one eye.

Inferior Oblique Inclusion. By far the most common cause of iatrogenic vertical deviation after horizontal muscle surgery is inferior oblique inclusion (not to be confused with inferior oblique adherence, discussed in the section "Inferior Oblique Adherence or Fat Adherence"). An inferior oblique inclusion is caused by inadvertent inclusion of the border of the inferior oblique when surgery is performed on the lateral rectus. It occurs most commonly with lateral rectus resection but can also occur after lateral rectus recession. Inferior oblique inclusion can be prevented by meticulous attention to freeing the attachments between the lateral rectus and the inferior oblique when performing surgery on the lateral rectus.

The patient with a new vertical deviation, either a hyperdeviation or a hypodeviation, after lateral rectus surgery should have the inferior border of the lateral rectus explored. If found, the inferior oblique inclusion should be freed and the

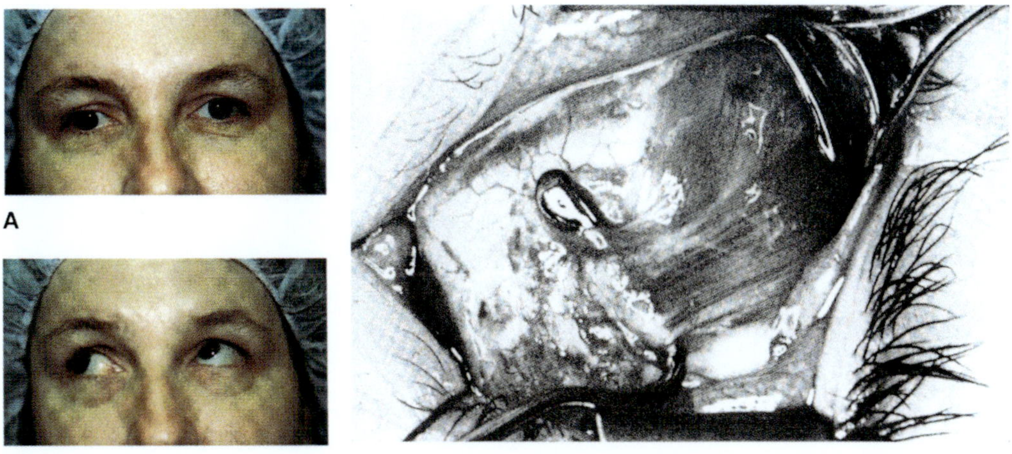

A

B

C

Figure 8–3. Inferior oblique inclusion. (*A*) Vertical deviation (right hypotropia) after lateral rectus resection. (*B*) Versions show limitation of elevation in the right eye, with secondary overaction of the left inferior oblique. (*C*) Intraoperative appearance of inclusion syndrome. Note that the right inferior oblique is dragged forward and attached to the new lateral rectus insertion.

muscle allowed to fall back into its normal anatomic position. Suturing the border of the inferior oblique to the globe will help prevent the new edges of the inferior oblique and lateral rectus from reattaching.

Despite freeing the inferior oblique inclusion into what appears to be a normal relationship with the lateral rectus, the induced vertical deviation can be disappointingly unaffected. Vertical rectus surgery is often needed either coincident to or after the inferior oblique surgery, and myectomy of the offending inferior oblique should be considered, depending on the preoperative deviation (Fig. 8–3).

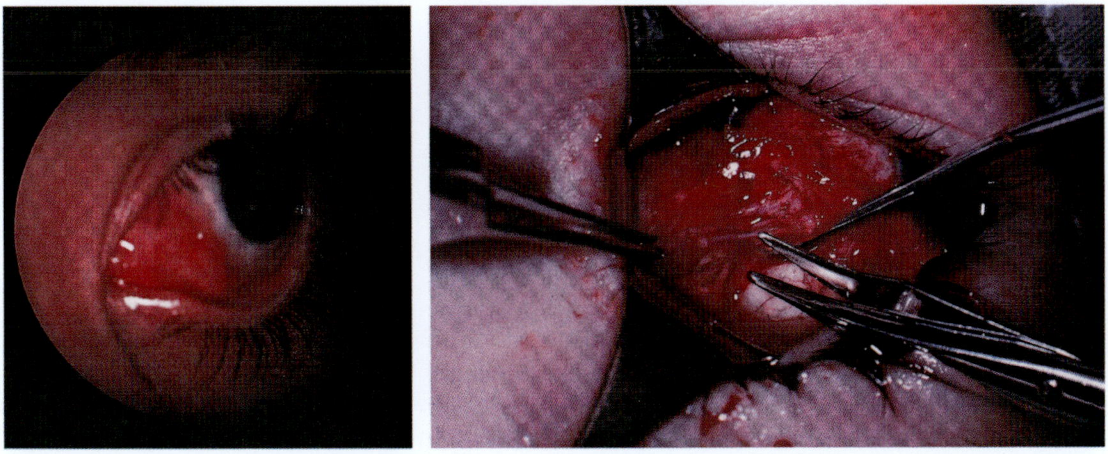

A

B

Figure 8–4. Fat adherence. (*A*) Fibro-fatty proliferation after violation of the extraconal fat pad around the medial rectus. (*B*) Intraoperative appearance of fat adherence. [Photos courtesy of Marshall M. Parks, MD]

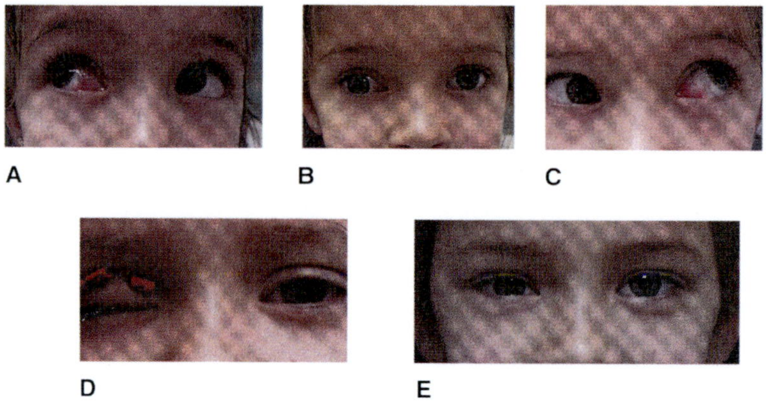

Figure 8–5. Traction sutures for treatment of inferior oblique adherence. (*A–C*) Appearance after surgery to weaken the right inferior oblique. Note the restriction to elevation of the right eye, worse in adduction. The patient had undergone three prior surgeries in an effort to improve the hypodeviation. (*D*) After extensive dissection and freeing of adhesions from the inferior globe, traction sutures are placed at the limbus, brought out through the upper lid, and left for 1 week. (*E*) Appearance 1 month postoperatively showing significant improvement in alignment.

Inferior Oblique Adherence, or Fat Adherence. Other causes of iatrogenic vertical deviation include other restrictive entities, such as adherence from fat-pad violation or inadvertent surgery on a vertical rectus muscle. Fat adherence is caused by violation of the extraconal fat pad, allowing fat to prolapse directly onto the globe surface. It may be evidenced by fatty proliferation under the conjunctiva, resulting in an unsightly scarred conjunctival surface (Fig. 8–4), although obvious external signs are not always present.

Many strategies to prevent readhesion of the orbital fat to the globe have been tried, including injection of corticosteroids intraoperatively and placement of muscle sleeves or sheets to separate the tissues, but none is very effective in preventing the restrictive process from recurring. A strategy that can be of some help is to use a traction suture to keep the globe in an exaggerated position for a week or more postoperatively while the initial healing takes place (Fig. 8–5).

REOPERATION FOR RESIDUAL OR CONSECUTIVE VERTICAL STRABISMUS

Reoperation on the Inferior Oblique. Most vertical strabismus involving the rectus muscles is related to paralytic or restrictive phenomena. Principles for these scenarios are discussed in Chapter 5, "Paralytic Strabismus," and Chapter 6, "Restrictive Strabismus." Reoperation involving previous oblique muscle surgery involves a different set of considerations and is discussed here.

The most commonly performed inferior oblique weakening procedures include recession, anterior transposition, myectomy, and denervation with extirpation (see Chapter 3, "Oblique Muscle Dysfunction").

Residual overaction after recession. Since the location of the inferior oblique is known, locating its new insertion in the inferior temporal quadrant should be possible. Great care must be exercised with the dissection to avoid lacerating posterior Tenon's capsule and causing inferior oblique adherence (fat adherence). Theoretically, the recession can be converted to a larger recession or an anterior transposition, but in most cases, converting the recession to a myectomy by transecting the muscle as it enters the sub-Tenon's space will effectively weaken the overacting muscle.

Residual overaction after anterior transposition. Anterior transposition is a very powerful weakening procedure and rarely results in recurrent overaction. When such overaction is apparent, it is likely due to a relative restriction to up gaze in the contralateral eye. Treatment aimed at relieving this restriction should be considered.

Residual overaction after myectomy. Three events can occur after a well-performed inferior oblique myectomy:

1. The inferior oblique will retract through Tenon's capsule and not reattach directly to the globe. Recurrent overaction is probably rare in this instance (Fig. 8–6A).
2. The inferior oblique will reattach to the globe somewhere in the inferior temporal quadrant. This is a very common occurrence but, depending on where on the globe the inferior oblique reattaches, it may or may not result in residual overaction (Fig. 8–6B).
3. The two cut ends of the inferior oblique will find each other and become reconnected through a fibrous connection. Depending on the length of the intervening fibrous band, this may or may not result in residual or recurrent overaction (Fig. 8–6C).

Traction testing of the inferior oblique is an indispensable tool when contemplating reoperation on an inferior oblique that has undergone previous myectomy.

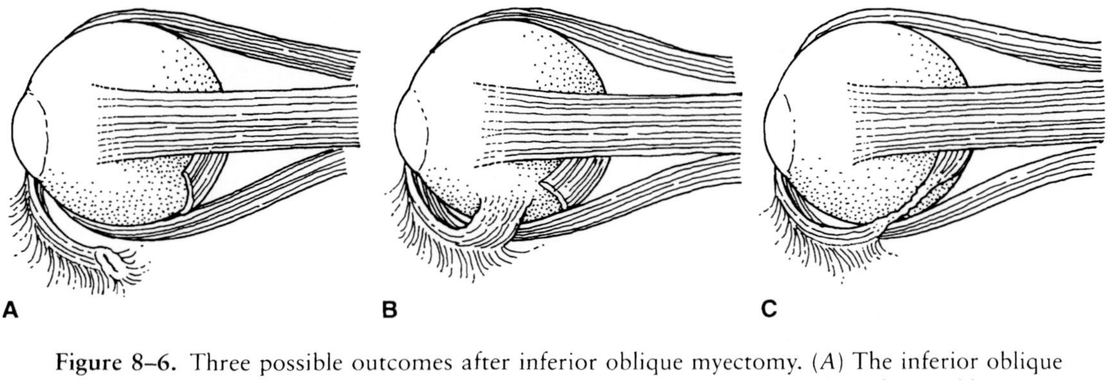

Figure 8–6. Three possible outcomes after inferior oblique myectomy. (*A*) The inferior oblique can retract through Tenon's capsule and not reattach to the globe. (*B*) The inferior oblique can reattach to the globe at a new location. (*C*) Two cut ends of the inferior oblique can reattach to each other through a fibrous band.

The technique is based on the exaggerated forced duction of the inferior oblique described by Guyton and is illustrated in Fig. 8–7.

If a distinct *band* of the inferior oblique is felt on the traction test, one of three events is responsible: the inferior oblique has reattached to the sclera, the two cut ends have reattached to each other, or the original myectomy was incomplete. With any scenario, careful exploration of the inferior temporal quadrant should reveal the responsible structure. At this point, the residual muscle in the sub-Tenon's space can be clamped, transected, and cauterized flush with the Tenon's penetration site (Fig. 8–8). Alternatively, if enough muscle can be recovered, the previous myectomy can be converted to an anterior transposition (Fig. 8–9).

If traction testing indicates no significant band of the inferior oblique, exploration of the inferior temporal quadrant looking for residual muscle will not be productive and can be avoided. Instead, attention should focus on the ipsilateral antagonist superior oblique or the yoke inferior rectus of the opposite eye.

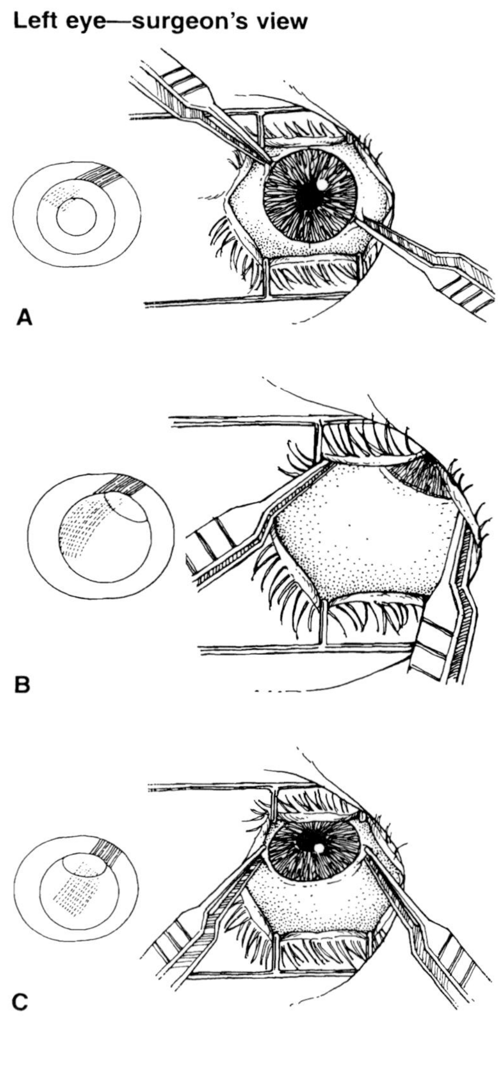

Figure 8–7. Technique of the inferior oblique traction test. The inset shows the relative position of the inferior oblique throughout the maneuver. (*A*) The eye is grasped at the limbus obliquely, for example, at the 4 o'clock and 10 o'clock positions on the left eye. (*B*) The eye is pushed down and in toward the inferonasal quadrant and then moved toward the inferotemporal quadrant. The eye will bump across the outstretched inferior oblique as it is pushed from the nasal to the temporal quadrant. (*C*) The eye can be rocked back and forth across the outstretched inferior oblique. The *band* felt on this test is wider and less distinct than on the analogous traction test of the superior oblique.

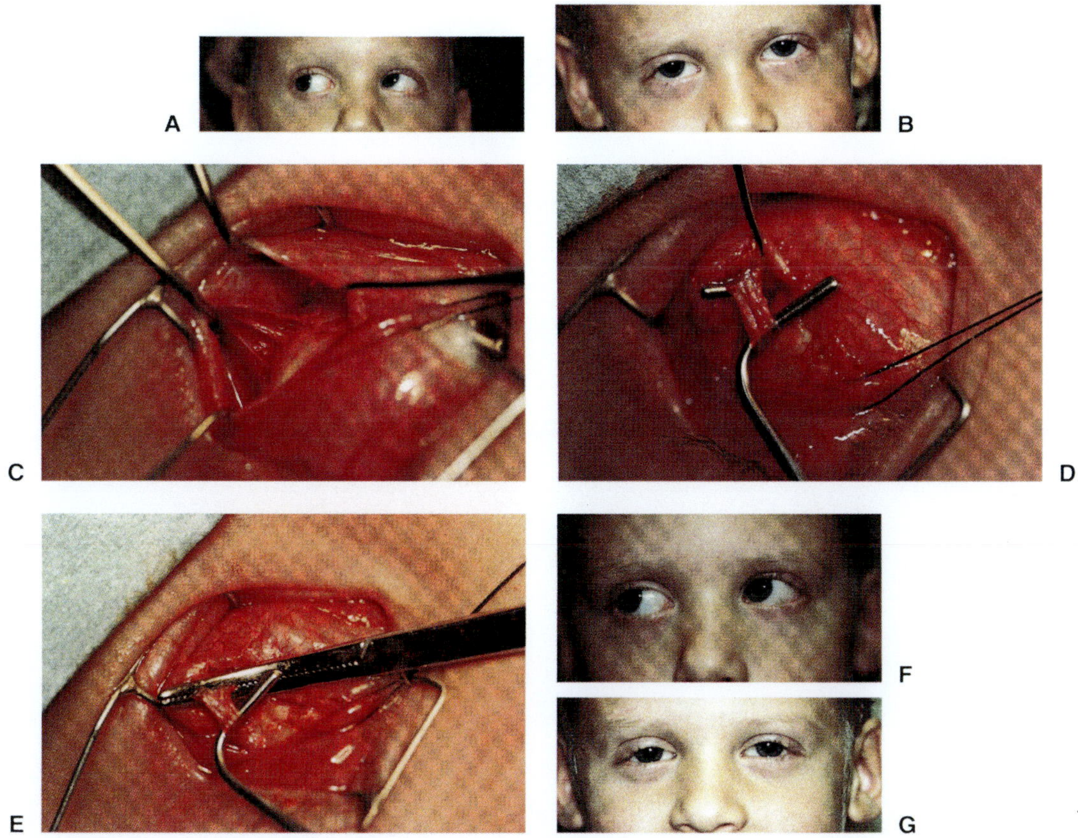

Figure 8–8. Inferior oblique overaction after myectomy. (*A*) Recurrent overaction of the left inferior oblique after myectomy for left superior oblique palsy. (*B*) Residual right head tilt is manifest. (*C*) Traction testing suggested the presence of a residual band of inferior oblique muscle. Intraoperative appearance of the inferior temporal quadrant showing adhesions to the globe. (*D*) Further dissection reveals the offending residual attachment of the inferior oblique to the globe. (*E*) Further myectomy is performed, clamping and then cutting the muscle flush with Tenon's penetration site. (*F*) Postoperative appearance showing no residual inferior oblique overaction. (*G*) Preoperative head tilt has been normalized.

COMMENT

Michael X. Repka, MD

This test should also be done intraoperatively (following the myectomy) at the time of the original inferior oblique surgery, as it can identify even a few fibers that may have been missed.

COMMENT

Gunter K. von Noorden, MD

In my experience, by far the most common cause of persistent upshoot in adduction after a myectomy of the inferior oblique muscle is failure to iden-

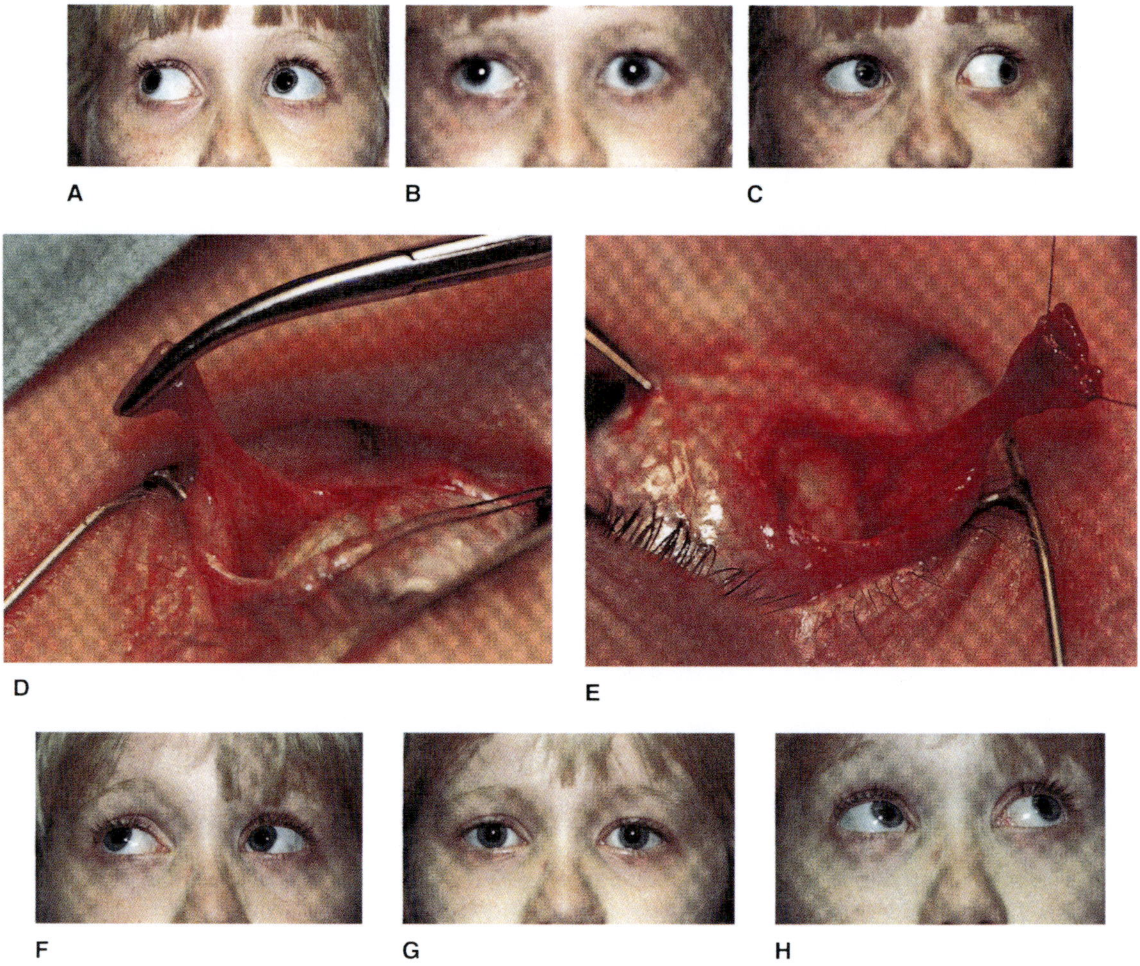

Figure 8–9. Inferior oblique overaction and dissociated vertical deviation after myectomy. (*A–C*) Preoperative appearance of manifest dissociated vertical deviation of the right eye and residual inferior oblique overaction greater in the right eye than in the left after bilateral myectomy. Traction testing suggested the presence of residual bands of inferior oblique muscle in both eyes. (*D,E*) Exploration of the inferior temporal quadrant reveals that the band was due to a fibrous connection joining two cut edges of the inferior oblique. Photographs show inferior obliques after disinsertion from the globe at their normal insertions. Note the pink skeletal muscle at the insertion as it transitions into a fibrous connective band that attaches to the proximal portion of the inferior oblique. The distal portion of muscle was excised; the remainder was reattached to the globe in its anterior transposition location. The identical situation was encountered in the opposite eye. (*F–H*) Postoperative appearance showing elimination of both inferior oblique overaction and manifest dissociated vertical deviation.

tify and engage the entire muscle on muscle hooks prior to the myectomy. A small bundle of posterior muscle fibers may slip off the tip of a hook, escape the myectomy, and suffice to cause persistent upshoot of the adducted eye, even after major portions of the muscle have been myectomized. The same is true of the failure to perform a complete tenectomy of the superior oblique muscle. Direct visualization of muscle or tendon prior to its exposure on muscle hooks will avoid this complication.

Residual overaction after denervation and extirpation. This powerful weakening procedure rarely results in residual overaction. If the muscle was securely pushed behind its Tenon's penetration site and the site sutured closed, there is unlikely to be a significant residual connection of the inferior oblique to the globe. Traction testing should confirm this, and attention can be turned to the ipsilateral superior oblique or contralateral inferior rectus to treat the residual hyperdeviation.

Underaction after weakening. Although relatively rare, inferior oblique underaction can occur after an inferior oblique weakening procedure (Fig. 8–10). The surgeon should first confirm that the underelevation of the affected eye is not due to a restrictive complication of the previous surgery.

As a practical matter, underaction after inferior oblique recession, myectomy, or extirpation cannot be reliably reversed by advancing or resecting the previously operated inferior oblique. A recession of the contralateral superior rectus will probably be more effective. The exception to this rule is underaction after inferior oblique anterior transposition. This procedure produces a relative restriction to up gaze, especially if performed unilaterally. The restriction or underaction can be improved by converting the anteriorization to a recession or myectomy.

Reoperation on the Superior Oblique.

Iatrogenic Brown syndrome. An overly aggressive tuck of the superior oblique will result in an iatrogenic Brown syndrome, manifested by underelevation of the affected eye in adduction (Fig. 8–11). If the underelevation is mild, it can be left untreated because the tuck will usually loosen somewhat with time. If the Brown syndrome is severe in the early postoperative period, the patient should be returned

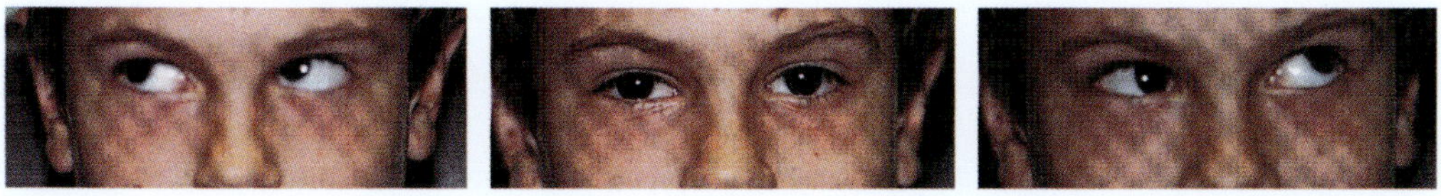

A B C

Figure 8–10. Inferior oblique underaction (right eye) after myectomy. The condition should be treated as case of inferior oblique palsy after confirming that the underaction is not due to a restrictive complication.

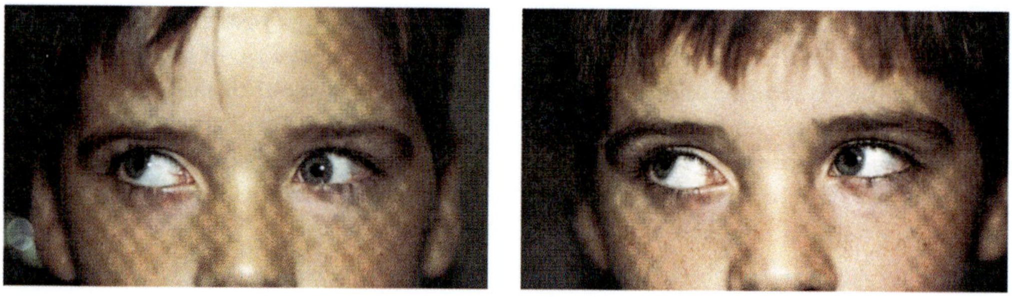

A B

Figure 8–11. Inferior oblique underaction due to iatrogenic Brown syndrome after superior oblique tuck. (*A*) Appearance after tuck. Mild Brown syndrome in the early postoperative period will usually resolve. (*B*) Appearance 2 months postoperatively showing improvement of elevation deficiency. With a more marked iatrogenic Brown syndrome, the tuck should be taken down surgically before permanent adhesions form in the tucked tendon. This complication can be avoided by careful traction testing intraoperatively to ensure that the tuck is not excessive.

to the operating room expeditiously to have the tuck taken down. Once adhesions have formed in the tucked tendon, freeing them can be difficult or impossible.

Residual underaction after tuck. Residual underaction of the superior oblique after a tuck can be remedied by further tucking of the tendon. A perhaps more common reason for persistent superior oblique underaction is ineffective weakening of the ipsilateral inferior oblique. The inferior oblique should be thoroughly weakened prior to further surgery to tighten the superior oblique tendon.

Residual overaction or up-gaze restriction after tenectomy. After a superior oblique tenectomy, recurrent overaction can be caused by one of three events:

1. The original tenectomy was incomplete.
2. The two cut ends of the tendon have rejoined.
3. The proximal end of the tendon has reattached to the globe. Reattachment of the superior oblique tendon to the globe is much less common than reattachment of the inferior oblique muscle to the globe after a myectomy.

Any of these three possibilities can be diagnosed by traction testing of the superior oblique. If a prominent band of superior oblique tendon is felt on traction testing, the area should be explored, the tendon identified (usually nasal to the superior rectus), and the connections severed. Traction testing must be repeated to ensure that all bands have been severed.

Residual or recurrent superior oblique overaction or, in the case of Brown syndrome, residual restriction to elevation caused by the superior oblique tendon after any weakening procedure on the superior oblique can be converted to a complete tenotomy. If a silicon spacer was previously used, replacing it with a larger spacer is impractical. Instead, the spacer should be removed and any adhesions of the superior oblique tendon to the globe freed.

Underaction after weakening. If clinically significant weakness of the superior oblique occurs after tenotomy or tenectomy of the superior oblique tendon, attempts to reestablish the integrity of the tendon can be made and sometimes successfully carried out, but may be futile. In such cases, the condition can be treated like a new case of superior oblique palsy (see Chapter 3, "Oblique Muscle Dysfunction"). In general, attention should be focused on appropriate weakening of the ipsilateral inferior oblique.

COMMENT

Marshall M. Parks, MD

Almost every time I have attempted surgically to find the cut ends of the superior oblique tendon, the attempt has been successful. I feel strongly that this is an important piece of information. The lesson is that the previously tenectomized tendons can be found, usually joined together with fibrous inelastic tissue, which should be excised prior to suturing the tendon ends together.

Suggested Readings

Ellis FD, Wasserman BN, Hidaji F: Selected surgical complications. In: Rosenbaum AL, Santiago AP, eds: *Clinical Strabismus Management: Principles and Surgical Techniques.* Philadelphia: WB Saunders Co; 1999, 539–551.

Helveston EM: *Surgical Management of Strabismus: An Atlas of Strabismus Surgery*, 4th ed. St Louis: CV Mosby Co; 1993.

Helveston EM, Alcorn DM, Ellis FD: Inferior oblique inclusion after lateral rectus surgery. *Graefes Arch Clin Exp Ophthalmol* 1988; 226:102–105.

Parks MM: Causes of the adhesive syndrome. In: *Symposium on Strabismus: Transactions of the New Orleans Academy of Ophthalmology.* St Louis: CV Mosby Co; 1978, 269–279.

Parks MM, Bloom JN: The "slipped" muscle. *Ophthalmology* 1979; 86:1389–1396.

Plager DA, Parks MM: Recognition and repair of the slipped rectus muscle. *J Pediatr Ophthalmol Strabismus* 1988; 25:270–274.

Plager DA, Parks MM: Recognition and repair of the "lost" rectus muscle: a report of 25 cases. *Ophthalmology* 1990; 97:131–136; discussion 136–137.

Rosenbaum AL, Santiago AP, eds: *Clinical Strabismus Management: Principles and Surgical Techniques.* Philadelphia: WB Saunders Co; 1999.

von Noorden GK: *Binocular Vision and Ocular Motility: Theory and Management of Strabismus*, 5th ed. St Louis: CV Mosby Co; 1996.

Index

Page numbers followed by f and t indicate figures and tables, respectively.

Printed and bound by CPI Group (UK) Ltd, Croydon, CR0 4YY